# WORKBOOK

# Maternal-Newborn Nursing

## A Family and Community-Based Approach

### SIXTH EDITION

**Marcia L. London**, RNC, MSN, NNP
*Associate Professor and Director*
*Neonatal Nurse Practitioner Program*
*Beth-El College of Nursing and Health Sciences at UCCS*
*Colorado Springs, Colorado*

**Patricia Wieland Ladewig**, RNC, PhD, NP
*Professor and Dean*
*School for Health Care Professions*
*Regis University*
*Denver, Colorado*

**Sally B. Olds**, RNC, MS, SANE
*Professor Emeritis*
*Colorado Springs, Colorado*

**Prentice Hall Health**
Upper Saddle River, New Jersey 07458

*We dedicate this book to our families—with love.*
David, Craig, and Matthew London
Tim, Ryan, and Erik Ladewig
Joe, Scott, and Allison Olds

Publisher: Julie Alexander
Editor-in-Chief: Cheryl Mehalik
Project Editor: Virginia Simione Jutson
Managing Editor: Wendy Earl
Associate Editor: Stephanie Kellogg
Publishing Assistants: Susan Teahan, Peggy Hammett
Production Supervisor: David Novak
Production Coordinator: Janet Vail
Director of Manufacturing and Production: Bruce Johnson
Manufacturing Buyer: Ilene Sanford
Cover Designer: Yvo Riezebos Design
Typesetting: Leigh McLellan
Printer/Binder: Courier
Cover: *I have found My Blue Flower,* quilted by Liesel Niesner and photographed by Charlotte de la Bedoyère.
Reproduced with kind permission of Search Press Ltd. © Search Press Ltd.

Previously published by Addison Wesley Nursing
A Division of the Benjamin/Cummings Publishing Company, Inc.
Menlo Park, California 94025

© 2000 by Prentice-Hall, Inc.
Upper Saddle River, New Jersey 07458

Printed in the United States of America

10 9 8 7 6 5 4 3 2

ISBN 0-8053-8074-4

Prentice-Hall International (UK) Limited, London
Prentice-Hall of Australia Pty. Limited, Sydney
Prentice-Hall Canada Inc., Toronto
Prentice-Hall Hispanoamericana, S.A., Mexico
Prentice-Hall India Private Limited, New Delhi
Prentice-Hall of Japan, Inc., Tokyo

# Preface

Maternal-newborn nurses are responsible for a complex, highly specialized body of knowledge related to the needs of the childbearing family, whether normal or at-risk. In recent years, that knowledge has expanded rapidly, as have the technology and complex ethical issues surrounding pregnancy and birth. In addition, these issues must be taught in a shorter period of time.

The *Maternal-Newborn Nursing Workbook* can assist in that effort by providing a concise, up-to-date review of maternal-newborn nursing theoretical content emphasizing application of the nursing process and critical thinking in clinical and community-based maternity settings. Selected women's health issues are also explored.

All major maternity texts include content related to the human reproductive system and to the antepartal, intrapartal, postpartal, and neonatal periods, although their sequences may vary. This workbook can also be used with most of the major maternity nursing texts, no matter what their organization. It is specifically designed to be used with *Maternal-Newborn Nursing: A Family and Community-Based Approach*, Sixth Edition by Olds, London, and Ladewig. The subjects follow the same sequence as in the textbook, although a few textbook chapters may be combined into one workbook topic. To assist the student, we have identified the pertinent corresponding text chapters at the beginning of each workbook topic. Internet resource information is also provided at the end of the topics. The workbook is appropriate for all types of nursing programs—baccalaureate, associate degree, and diploma. Nurses involved in refresher courses or just entering this specialty area will also find it helpful. Practicing nurses may find it helpful, too, especially in assessment and critical clinical decision making.

## Features of This Edition

By its very nature, maternal-newborn nursing is community-based nursing. Only a brief portion of the entire pregnancy and birth is spent in a birthing center or hospital. Moreover, because of changes in practice, even women with high-risk pregnancies are receiving more care in their homes and in the community and spending less time in hospital settings.

The provision of nursing care in community-based settings is a driving force in health care today and, consequently, questions on community-based care are included throughout this workbook.

This workbook also emphasizes the application and synthesis of an expanding research-based, maternal-newborn nursing clinical knowledge. Because we learn best through active learning, we have provided critical thinking scenarios to further develop your critical decision-making and prioritizing skills. Critical thinking challenge situations are presented, and the student is asked to prioritize nursing actions. Critical thinking in practice sequences have been developed for selected normal and complication chapters to provide realistic clinical practice situations. Clinical data are presented, and the student is guided through the decision-making process for a particular situation.

Because we believe that sound clinical judgment develops from theoretical knowledge, research, and practical experience, most of the items in this workbook are based on clinical situations. Recognizing the rich cultural heritage of our diverse population, many of these client situations include ethnic families.

Working with the childbearing family is an intensely rewarding interactive nursing experience. The review of these clinical experiences and/or a personal childbearing experience increases our understanding of the universal childbirth/parenting experience. We have provided the student with opportunities in the *Reflections* feature to revisit and ponder those experiences.

Some of the questions are related to factual material, and students can verify their answers easily in the provided answer section at the end of the workbook. However, for those questions that require synthesis and more application, we have established a critical thinking dialogue with the student to assist in self-assessment. In addition we have provided the pertinent pages in the textbook for the student for those more complex questions.

## Clarification of Terms

Although we recognize that the men in nursing are becoming more involved in the provision of maternity care, women are still the major care providers. Therefore, whenever possible, we have avoided sexist pronouns in referring to the nurse. When this was not possible, we have used the female pronoun.

By the same token, we appreciate the fact that the individual who is most significant to the pregnant woman may be her husband, the father of the child, another family member, or simply a good friend, male or female. Thus we have provided both traditional "husband-wife" situations, and situations involving other support persons.

## Acknowledgments

First, we would like to recognize the students who reviewed the previous edition of this workbook. They approached their review seriously and provided many candid comments. They identified material that they felt was unclear and added valuable suggestions that enhance this edition.

We thank the nurse educators and practicing nurses who reviewed this material and offered their suggestions and comments. Their input helped us focus on the most pertinent material and offered a broader perspective.

Last but not least, we thank our families. We recognize the countless ways that they continue to help us and the sacrifices that they make as we pursue this other love. Women can accomplish any goal; however, combining marriage, family, intellectual challenges, and a career requires a supportive, adaptive, responsive family. Each of us is blessed with such a family. We love them.

M.L.L.
P.W.L.
S.B.O.

# Contents

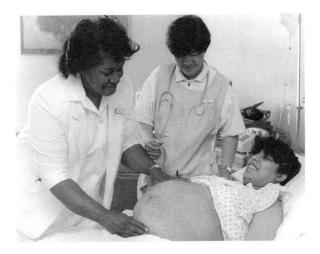

TOPIC

# 1 Contemporary Maternal-Newborn Care

The broad scope of maternity nursing offers a variety of professional opportunities and greatly increases the quality of care available to childbearing families. Nurses today draw on their educational and professional expertise and also use family and statistical data in planning and providing care.

This topic provides an introduction to the current roles of maternity nurses. It then focuses on pertinent statistical data. The latter portion of the topic focuses on client teaching.

This topic corresponds to Chapters 1 and 2 in the sixth edition of *Maternal-Newborn Nursing: A Family and Community-Based Approach*.

## Contemporary Childbirth

1. List at least three changes that have occurred in childbirth practices over the past 25 years.

   a.

   b.

   c.

2. Identify the main provisions of the Newborns' and Mothers' Health Protection Act of 1996, which took effect in 1998.

# Nursing Roles

3.   Maternity nurses function in a variety of roles in providing care to childbearing families. Define each of the following roles with emphasis on educational background and scope of function:

   a.   Professional nurse

   b.   Clinical nurse specialist (CNS)

   c.   Nurse practitioner (NP)

   d.   Certified nurse-midwife (CNM)

4.   Which of the following would be most qualified to provide prenatal, intrapartal, postpartal, and newborn care for the low-risk childbearing woman?
   a.   Acute-care clinical nurse specialist
   b.   Certified nurse-midwife
   c.   Lay midwife
   d.   Obstetric or women's health care nurse practitioner

# Community-Based Nursing Care

5.   The three areas of focus of primary care include _____, _____, and _____.

6.   Primary care is best provided in a _____ setting.

7.   Identify two purposes of home care.

   a.

   b.

## Standards of Care

8.  Discuss the standards of care that shape maternal-newborn nursing.

9.  Briefly describe the Human Genome Project and its implications for health care.

---

**REFLECTIONS**

There are many difficult ethical issues affecting the childbearing woman and family today. What do you think the most difficult issue will be for you in your maternal-newborn nursing course?

_____

_____

_____

_____

_____

_____

## Descriptive Statistics

10.  Define the following terms:

    a.  Birth rate

    b.  Infant mortality rate

    c.  Neonatal mortality

    d.  Maternal mortality

11.  Identify factors that may contribute to the decrease in the maternal mortality rate.

12.  Perinatal mortality is a combination of
    a.  infant death rate and neonatal mortality.
    b.  fetal death rate and infant death rate.
    c.  neonatal mortality and postneonatal mortality.
    d.  fetal death rate and neonatal mortality.

## Client Teaching

13.  Briefly summarize the impact of each of the following issues on client teaching.

    a.  Political issues

b.   Sociocultural issues

c.   Education and experience

d.   Technologic issues

---

## REFLECTIONS

Consider a situation in which you have either done some client teaching you feel was very successful or a situation that you believe was not very successful. Then answer the following questions:

1.   What assessments did you make about the individual's (or family's) needs?

2.   Did you involve the individual or family in developing the teaching session? If so, how?

3.   In implementing your teaching plan, what teaching strategies did you use?

→

*Reflections, continued*

4. Why did you select those strategies?

5. What factors led to the success or lack of success of your teaching?

6. If you could do it again, would you change anything? If so, what?

## Internet Resources

**http://www. guideline.gov**
Health care professionals will find recently published clinical practice guidelines and related abstracts of maternal-newborn care on the National Guidelines Clearinghouse web site.

# 2 Women's Health Care

A woman's health care needs change throughout her life and may be influenced by a variety of factors, such as her age, her family history, her plans for childbearing, her sexual activity, and any abnormal findings that develop. This topic focuses on selected social issues, health care issues, and gynecologic problems. It concludes with a discussion of violence against women.

This topic corresponds to Chapters 3, 4, and 5 in the sixth edition of *Maternal-Newborn Nursing: A Family and Community-Based Approach*.

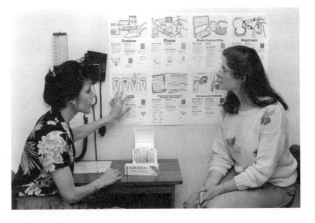

## The Role of the Nurse in Menstrual Counseling

Match the definitions listed on the right with the correct terms below.

1. _____ Amenorrhea     a. Abnormally short menstrual cycle

2. _____ Hypomenorrhea     b. Absence of menses

3. _____ Menorrhagia     c. Excessive menstrual flow

4. _____ Dysmenorrhea     d. Bleeding between periods

5. _____ Hypermenorrhea     e. Painful menses

6. _____ Metrorrhagia     f. Abnormally long menstrual cycle

7. Discuss premenstrual syndrome (PMS) with regard to etiology, signs and symptoms, and treatment. Include information on self-care measures women with PMS might employ.

## REFLECTIONS

Some women view menstruation as a normal, even welcome, part of life; some women view it as a minor annoyance; some women are embarrassed by it; others consider it a "curse" and hate it. Take a few moments to explore your views on menstruation. Try to identify some of the factors that have influenced your attitudes about it.

_____

_____

_____

_____

_____

_____

_____

## Contraceptive Methods

For each of the methods of contraception listed below, select the appropriate mechanism of action from the list on the right.

8. _____ Condom             a.  Prevents ovulation

9. _____ Norplant           b.  Prevents transport of sperm to the ovum

10. _____ Diaphragm

11. _____ Depo-Provera

12. _____ Oral contraceptive

13.  When using a diaphragm, the woman should use additional spermicide before intercourse if

   more than (a) _____ hours have elapsed since the diaphragm was inserted. She should

   leave the diaphragm in place for at least (b) _____ hours after intercourse.

14.    Marcella Heidegger has two children by a previous marriage. She has just begun seeing a man and asks you if the IUD would be a good contraceptive method if they become sexually involved. How would you respond?

15.    The male sterilization procedure is called (a) _____; female sterilization is

called (b) _____.

16.    An estrogen-related side effect of oral contraceptives is

    a.    acne.

    b.    decreased libido.

    c.    hirsutism.

    d.    hypertension.

# Gynecologic Screening Procedures

How often should each of the following screening procedures be performed?

17.    Breast self-examination _____

18.    Mammogram (woman age 32 at low risk for breast cancer) _____

19.    Mammogram (woman age 53) _____

20.    Pap smear (sexually active woman age 16) _____

21.    Pap smear (woman age 32) _____

22.    Identify three components of a pelvic examination:

    a.

    b.

    c.

23.    In performing a breast self-examination (BSE), why should a woman visually inspect her breasts with her arms in a variety of positions?

24.    Explain the procedure for breast self-examination.

25.    Which of the following findings during breast self-examination should a woman report to her health care provider?

a.    Difference in size between the breasts

b.    Silver-colored striae

c.    Symmetrical venous pattern

d.    Thickened skin with enlarged pores

# Menopause

26.    Mrs Joan Sanchez, age 50, has been coming to this office for her gynecologic exams for the past 7 years. Last year, she mentioned some irregularity in her periods. During her annual physical exam and Pap smear, she tells you that her periods have been more irregular and her last period was about 3 months ago. In addition, she has been experiencing difficulty sleeping; a sense of heat rising over her chest, neck, and face; increased perspiration; and palpitations.

You identify that Mrs Sanchez is entering menopause. In your counseling session, what information about self-care measures can you provide?

27.    **Critical Thinking Challenge:** The following situation has been included to challenge your critical thinking. Read the situation and then answer the question "yes" or "no."

Yvonne Swenson, age 52, is being seen for her annual examination. Her history reveals that she is a slender woman of Swedish ancestry who completed menopause at age 46. She does not drink alcohol but does smoke three-fourths of a pack of cigarettes per day. She has two children.

**Is Yvonne at increased risk of developing osteoporosis?**

Yes _____                           No _____

Explain your answer:

28.    In women who have a uterus and who are on hormone replacement therapy (HRT), the estrogen is opposed by giving (a) _____ for all or part of the cycle to prevent the increased risk of developing (b) _____ .

29.    Which of the following is a risk factor for osteoporosis?

a.    African American race

b.    Late onset of menopause

c.    Multiparity

d.    Thin and small-boned build

## Disorders of the Breast

Match the conditions below with the best description:

30. _____ Fibroadenoma

31. _____ Galactorrhea

32. _____ Duct ectasia

a. Nipple discharge

b. Excessive milk production in a lactating woman

c. Tumor growing in the terminal portion of a breast duct

d. Common, benign solid breast tumor

e. Inflammation of the ducts behind the nipple

33.   Your client experiences discomfort cyclically because of fibrocystic breast disease and asks if there are self-care measures she can use to alleviate her discomfort. What advice would you give her?

## Gynecologic Disorders

34.   The three most common symptoms of endometriosis are

  a. _____    b. _____    c. _____

35.   In the office where you work as a nurse, one of the women being treated for endometriosis is going to begin taking danazol. You assess her knowledge level and find that she has only a vague understanding of the medication. You formulate the nursing diagnosis *Knowledge Deficit* related to lack of information about the medication danazol. Based on this nursing diagnosis, what information would you give her about the drug?

36. A primary side effect of danazol (Danocrine) is
    a. dry, flaky skin.
    b. hirsutism.
    c. increased libido.
    d. weight loss.

37. Your client asks you about health practices she can follow to help her avoid developing toxic shock syndrome (TSS). What recommendations would you make?

Match the characteristic vaginal discharge listed on the right with the correct type of vaginitis.

38. _____ Bacterial vaginosis          a. Greenish-white and frothy

39. _____ Trichomoniasis               b. Thick, white, curdy

40. _____ Vulvovaginal candidiasis     c. Gray, milky

41. The presence of clue cells on a wet mount preparation is indicative of
    a. bacterial vaginosis.
    b. chlamydia.
    c. trichomoniasis.
    d. vulvovaginal candidiasis.

For each of the infections listed below, select the appropriate antibiotic treatment from the list on the right for a woman who is not pregnant.

42. _____ Chlamydia                     a. Benzathine penicillin G

43. _____ Gonorrhea                     b. Butoconazole

44. _____ Syphilis                      c. Ceftriaxone

45. _____ Vulvovaginal candidiasis      d. Doxycycline

46.    **Critical Thinking in Practice:** The following action sequence is designed to help you think through clinical problems. Read the sequence below, then fill in the appropriate boxes in the flowchart that follows.

Imagine you work as a registered nurse in a women's health clinic. It is your responsibility to interview women initially and obtain data on the purpose of their visit. You also do health teaching. You do not do pelvic examinations. Nita Trujillo, a client at the clinic, tells you she is there today because she has had marked itching of her vulva and vagina. She states, "It itches so bad that I've scratched it raw and made it worse." She tells you she has never had a vaginal infection before and has not been sexually active for three months. She says that she has had no symptoms of a urinary tract infection although it does burn when the urine touches the excoriated skin.

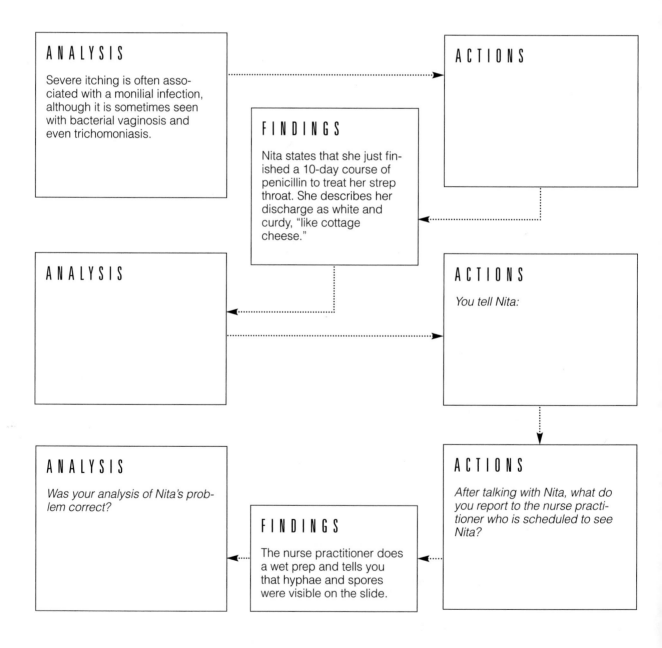

**ANALYSIS**

Severe itching is often associated with a monilial infection, although it is sometimes seen with bacterial vaginosis and even trichomoniasis.

**FINDINGS**

Nita states that she just finished a 10-day course of penicillin to treat her strep throat. She describes her discharge as white and curdy, "like cottage cheese."

**ACTIONS**

**ANALYSIS**

**ACTIONS**

You tell Nita:

**ANALYSIS**

Was your analysis of Nita's problem correct?

**FINDINGS**

The nurse practitioner does a wet prep and tells you that hyphae and spores were visible on the slide.

**ACTIONS**

After talking with Nita, what do you report to the nurse practitioner who is scheduled to see Nita?

47.    Marcy D'Angelo, diagnosed with trichomoniasis, has been given prescriptions for metronidazole for her and her partner. In addition to general teaching about the medication, what specific warning should you give Marcy?

48.    The greatest long-term problem caused by pelvic inflammatory disease (PID) is _____.

49.    Compare cystitis and pyelonephritis.

| | Cystitis | Pyelonephritis |
|---|---|---|
| Signs and symptoms | | |
| Therapy | | |
| Implications | | |
| Client education | | |

# Social Issues

50.    What proportion of children living in female-headed households are classified as living in poverty?

    a.    One in ten

    b.    One in eight

    c.    One in five

    d.    One in three

51. Summarize the major components of the Personal Responsibility and Work Opportunity Reconciliation Act.

52. Elderly women are at increased risk of poverty. Identify at least four factors contributing to this problem.

    a.

    b.

    c.

    d.

53. Discuss the impact of poverty on health care.

Environmental hazards in the workplace are often major concerns for women. Two agencies, OSHA and NIOSH, have been established to address the issue of environmental hazards in the workplace.

54. What does OSHA stand for? _____

55. What is the primary focus of OSHA?

56.   What does NIOSH stand for? _____

57.   What is the primary focus of NIOSH?

58.   Compare child abuse to elder abuse.

# Violence Against Women

59.   Define *domestic violence*.

60.   Estimates suggest that _____ in _____ women will be assaulted by a partner at some time in the woman's life.

61.   Because female partner abuse is so common, many experts advocate universal screening of all female clients whenever they are seen by a health care provider. In caring for a nonpregnant woman, what are the two questions you should ask to screen for abuse?

   a.


   b.

62.    If the woman is pregnant, what additional question should you ask?

63.    You are caring for a woman who is abused, but she does not feel able to leave the situation. You encourage her to make an exit plan for herself and her children. What should be part of an exit plan?

Match the definitions on the right with the type of rape they best describe.

64.    _____ Anger rape

a.    Assailant is known to the victim; previously the relationship was nonviolent

65.    _____ Confidence rape

b.    Assailant wishes to feel dominant and typically uses only the force necessary to subdue his victim

66.    _____ Power rape

c.    Attack is used to express feelings of rage and is often brutal and degrading

67.    _____ Sadistic rape

d.    Planned assault characterized by torture, mutilation, and often murder

68.    Briefly describe the Sexual Assault Nurse Examiner (SANE) Program.

69.   **Memory Check:** Define the following abbreviations.

a.   BBT                          e.   FBD

b.   BSE                          f.   PID

c.   CDC                          g.   STD

d.   D&C                          h.   UTI

# Internet Resources

**http://www.vh.org**
Through the University of Iowa, the Virtual Hospital web site offers a digital health sciences library, which provides obstetric and gynecologic information.

**http://www.womens-health.com**
The Women's Health Interactive web site includes a Frequently Asked Questions (FAQs) section that provides information on menstrual disorders, endometriosis, cancer, fibroids, and sexually transmitted diseases.

# 3 The Reproductive System

Puberty represents a major milestone in a young person's life. Secondary sex characteristics develop, the reproductive organs mature, and the person becomes capable of procreation. This topic reviews the female and male reproductive systems and the menstrual cycle, and reinforces the knowledge base from which maternity nursing care is derived.

This topic corresponds to Chapter 6 in the sixth edition of *Maternal-Newborn Nursing: A Family and Community-Based Approach*.

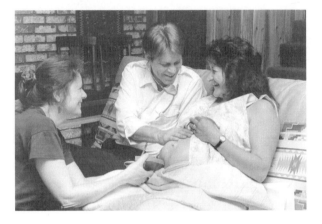

## Puberty

### REFLECTIONS

Puberty comes as a surprise to some, whereas others are well prepared. How well prepared were you for the experience? What might you do or have you done to prepare your children for puberty? What are your memories of going through puberty?

_____

_____

_____

_____

_____

_____

# Female Reproductive System

Match the external genitalia structure with its function or characteristics during the childbearing period.

1. _____ Clitoris

    a.  Produces smegma that has a sexually stimulating odor

2. _____ Labia minora

    b.  Protects pelvic bones, especially during coitus

3. _____ Mons pubis

    c.  Rich in sebaceous glands that lubricate and provide bactericidal secretions

4. _____ Paraurethral (Skene's) glands

    d.  Secretes clear thick mucus that enhances sperm viability and motility

5. _____ Perineal body

    e.  Secretions lubricate vaginal vestibule to facilitate sexual intercourse

6. _____ Vulvovaginal (Bartholin's) glands

    f.  Site of episiotomy and lacerations

7. Figure 3–1 below shows the female internal reproductive organs. Identify the structures that are indicated.

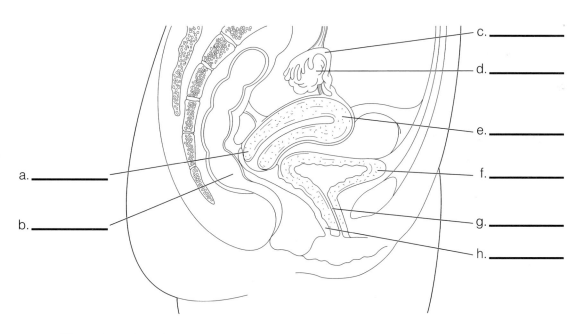

c. _____
d. _____
e. _____
f. _____
g. _____
h. _____
a. _____
b. _____

**Figure 3–1**  Female internal reproductive organs.

8. Briefly discuss the function(s) of the vagina.

9.  What factors can alter the vagina's pH and decrease its self-cleansing action?

10. Label the uterine structures indicated in Figure 3–2.

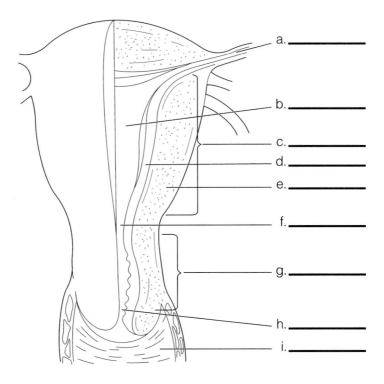

a._____

b._____

c._____

d._____

e._____

f._____

g._____

h._____

i._____

**Figure 3–2** Anatomy of the uterus.

11. The figure-eight pattern of the middle layer of uterine muscle fibers
    a.  causes cervical effacement.
    b.  constricts large uterine blood vessels when the fibers contract.
    c.  forms sphincters at fallopian tube attachment sites.
    d.  maintains the effects of uterine contractions during labor.

12. Briefly describe the function of the endometrium.

13. Identify three functions of the cervical mucosa.

    a.

    b.

    c.

14.    A group of adolescents is waiting for pregnancy tests in a clinic. One of the girls asks about infections. The nurse explains that certain body functions protect the female from infection of the reproductive organs. Which of the following protects the female from infection of the reproductive organs?

    a.    Alkaline pH and smegma secreted from the clitoris

    b.    Acidic pH and bacteriostatic cervical mucosa

    c.    Neutral pH of 7.5 and bactericidal secretions of the labia minora

    d.    pH of 4 to 5 and secretions of the Skene's ducts

15.    Identify the location and function of each of the following uterine ligaments:

| Ligament | Location | Function |
|---|---|---|
| Broad ligaments | | |
| Round ligaments | | |
| Cardinal ligaments | | |
| Infundibulopelvic ligament | | |
| Uterosacral ligaments | | |
| Ovarian ligaments | | |

16.    What are the primary functions of the fallopian tubes?

17.   In relation to the fallopian tubes, what is the purpose or significance of each of the following?

   a.   Fimbria


   b.   Isthmus


   c.   Ampulla


   d.   Muscular layer


   e.   Nonciliated goblet cells of the mucosa


   f.   Tubal cilia


18.   Briefly describe the function of the three layers (tunica albuginea, cortex, medulla) of the ovary.


19.   What is (are) the primary function(s) of the ovaries?

20.    Label the following pelvic bones and supporting ligaments in Figure 3–3.

Sacrum                  Symphysis pubis        Sacroiliac ligament      Sacrotuberous ligament

Left innominate bone    Right sacroiliac joint Sacrospinous ligament    Coccyx

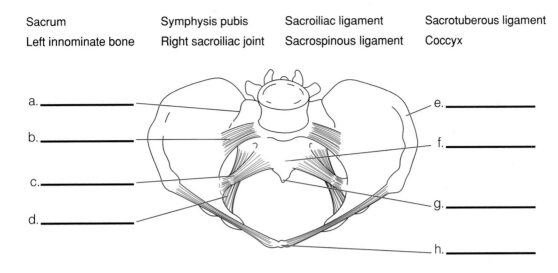

a._____

b._____

c._____

d._____

e._____

f._____

g._____

h._____

**Figure 3–3**   Bony pelvis with ligaments.

21.    Figure 3–4 focuses on the muscles of the pelvic floor. Label the following structures:

Vagina                       Iliococcygeus muscle       External anal sphincter

Bulbospongiosus muscle       Ischial tuberosity         Urogenital diaphragm

Gluteus maximus muscle       Adductor longus muscle

Ischiocavernosus muscle      Pubococcygeus muscle

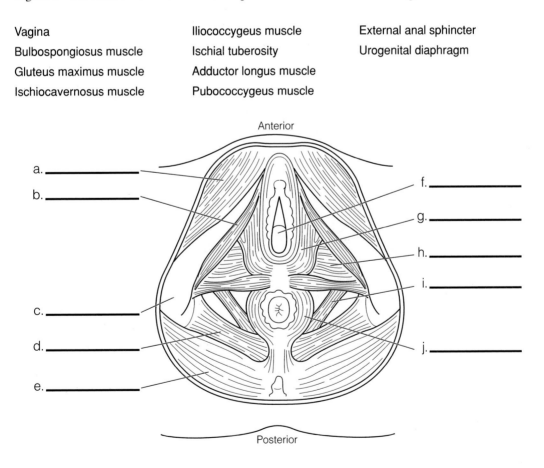

Anterior

a._____

b._____

c._____

d._____

e._____

f._____

g._____

h._____

i._____

j._____

Posterior

**Figure 3–4**   Muscles of the pelvic floor.

22.   The major muscle group that forms the pelvic diaphragm is the _____ .

23.   Define each of the following terms and briefly identify its implications for childbearing:

   a.   False pelvis

   b.   True pelvis

   c.   Pelvic inlet

   d.   Pelvic outlet

24.   In Figure 3–5, label the false pelvis, true pelvis, pelvic inlet, and pelvic outlet.

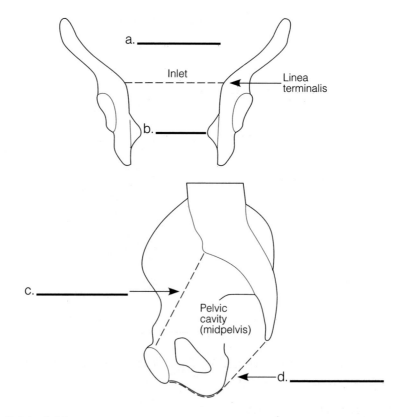

**Figure 3–5**   Pelvic divisions.

25.   Label the major structures of the breast in Figure 3–6.

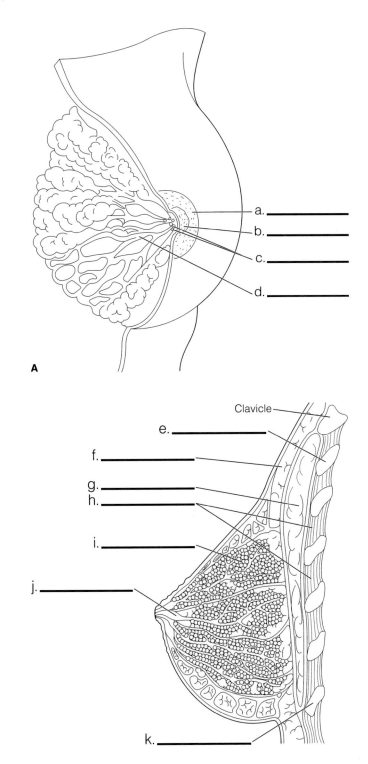

a. _____

b. _____

c. _____

d. _____

Clavicle

e. _____

f. _____

g. _____
h. _____

i. _____

j. _____

k. _____

**Figure 3–6**   Anatomy of the breast. **A** Anterior view of partially dissected left breast.
**B** Sagittal section.

26.   What is the primary function of the tubercles of Montgomery?

27.   What portion of the breast contains the cuboidal epithelial cells that secrete the components of milk?

   a.   Alveoli

   b.   Ducts

   c.   Lactiferous sinuses

   d.   Lobules

# Female Reproductive Cycle (FRC)

28.   The female reproductive cycle is made up of two interrelated cycles that occur simultaneously: the

   (a) _____ cycle and the (b) _____ cycle.

29.   For each of the following hormones involved in ovulation and menstruation, state the source of secretion and the primary function(s).

| Hormone | Source | Function(s) |
| --- | --- | --- |
| Estrogen | | |
| Progesterone | | |
| Follicle-stimulating hormone (FSH) | | |
| Gonadotropin-releasing hormone (GnRH) | | |
| Luteinizing hormone (LH) | | |
| Prostaglandins (PGE and PGF$_{2a}$) | | |

30.  A girl waiting for a pregnancy test asks the nurse which hormone causes ovulation to occur. The nurse explains that about 18 hours after the peak production of _____, ovulation occurs.

   a.   estrogen

   b.   FSH (follicle-stimulating hormone)

   c.   LH (luteinizing hormone)

   d.   progesterone

31.  The nurse asks the girl to identify the hormone responsible for enhancing development of the graafian follicle and rebuilding the endometrium. The right answer would be

   a.   estrogen.

   b.   FSH–RH (follicle-stimulating hormone–releasing hormone).

   c.   GnRH (gonadotropin-releasing hormone).

   d.   LHRH (luteinizing hormone–releasing hormone).

32.  Describe the process of ovulation and the related changes in the ovarian follicle.

33.  Briefly describe the changes that occur in each of the following during the various phases of the menstrual cycle.

   a.   Endometrium

   b.   Cervical mucosa

34.   Label the following components of the menstrual cycle in Figure 3–7.

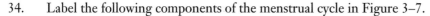

| Menstrual | Secretory | Follicular | Estrogen |
| Proliferative | Ischemic | Luteal | Progesterone |

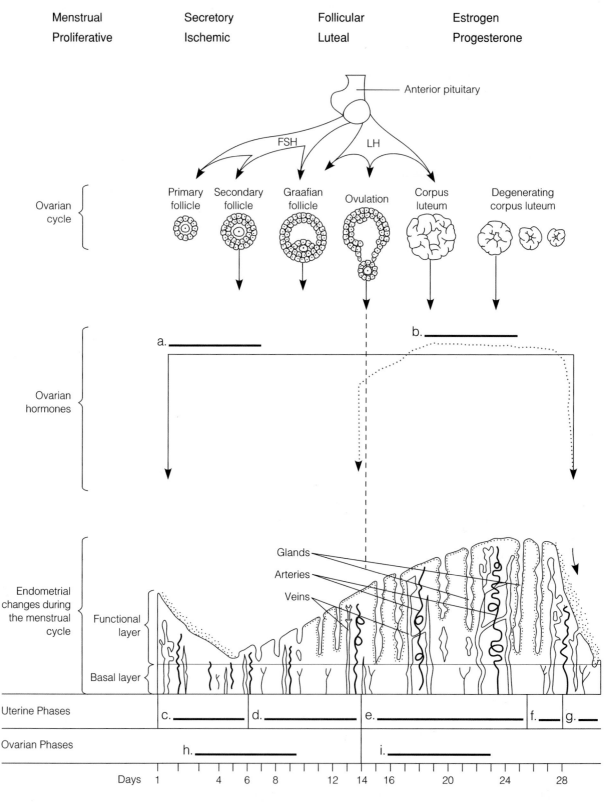

**Figure 3–7**   Female reproductive cycle: Interrelationships of hormones and the four phases of the uterine cycle and two phases of the ovarian cycle.

35.    How would you explain the process of menstruation to a group of adolescents?

# Male Reproductive System

36.    The most important purpose for the location of the scrotum is to

    a.    maintain temperature lower than that of the body.

    b.    produce sperm near the point of ejaculation.

    c.    protect the testes and sperm from the effects of the prostate.

    d.    provide room for the convoluted seminiferous tubules.

37.    Complete the following sentences using the words related to the male reproductive structures and functions listed below.

| | | |
|---|---|---|
| Bulbourethral (Cowper's) glands | penis | seminal vesicles |
| epididymides | prostate gland | testis |
| ejaculatory duct | Sertoli's cells | testes |
| Leydig's cells | seminal fluid (semen) | vas deferens |

The visible male reproductive organs include the (a) _____ and the scrotum. The primary function of the scrotum is protection; it contains the (b) _____,

(c) _____, and (d) _____: the male internal reproductive structures.

Each (e) _____ produces testosterone via the (f) _____, which houses the seminiferous tubules and immature sperm. Maturation of sperm occurs in the

(g) _____, the storage area for mature spermatozoa. Seminiferous tubules

contain (h) _____ cells that nourish and protect the spermatocytes.

The (i) _____ secretes fluids high in fructose and prostaglandins that

nourish sperm and increase their motility. The vas deferens and the duct of a seminal vesicle

unite to form a short tube called the (j) _____, which passes through the

prostate gland and terminates in the urethra. The (k) _____ gland secretes

thin, alkaline fluid containing calcium and other substances that counteract the acidity of ductus

and seminal vesicle secretions. The prostate gland secretes substances in the (l) _____

_____. The (m) _____ glands secrete viscous, alkaline fluid rich in

mucoproteins, which neutralize the acid in the male urethra and the vagina.

38.    **Memory Check:** Define the following abbreviations.

a.   FRC                                  c.   GnRH


b.   FSH                                  d.   LH

# 4 Conception, Fetal Development, and Special Reproductive Issues

The conception and development of a new human being is a never-ending source of awe and fascination.

This topic begins with a review of the process of conception. It then considers implantation, placental functioning, and fetal development. Factors that may influence fetal development are explored, with special emphasis on the impact of maternal medications. Also discussed are the issues of infertility and the impact of genetics on reproduction. Most couples who want children are able to have them with little difficulty. In some instances, couples may be unable to fulfill their dream of having a baby because of special reproductive issues.

This topic corresponds to Chapters 7 and 8 in the sixth edition of *Maternal-Newborn Nursing: A Family and Community-Based Approach*.

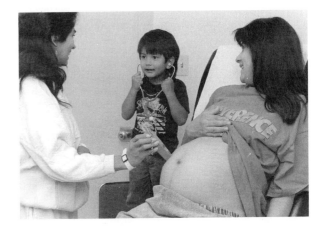

## Cellular Division

1. Briefly compare mitosis and meiosis.

2. The optimal time for fertilization to occur is (a) _____ hours after ovulation of the ovum and (b) _____ hours after ejaculation.

3. Each sperm and ovum has (a) _____ chromosomes. When sperm and ovum are united, the resulting normal newborn has (b) _____ chromosomes.

4. The (a) _____ chromosome determines the sex of the child. The (b) _____ carries this chromosome.

5.   Fertilization occurs in the

   a.   cervix.

   b.   fallopian tube.

   c.   ovary.

   d.   uterus.

6.   Briefly describe the process of fertilization.

7.   Describe the two processes that the sperm undergoes in order to fertilize the ovum.

   a.

   b.

## Cellular Multiplication and Implantation

The zygote continually develops as it travels through the fallopian tube to its site of implantation in the uterus. Match each of the following terms with the appropriate description.

8.   _____ Cleavage          a.   Period of rapid cellular division

9.   _____ Blastomeres       b.   Outer layer of cells that replaces the zona pellucida

10.  _____ Morula            c.   Small developing mass of cells held together by zona pellucida

11.  _____ Blastocyst        d.   Solid ball of cells

12.  _____ Trophoblasts      e.   Inner solid mass of cells after cavity has formed

13.  Implantation occurs about (a) _____ to (b) _____ days after fertilization. Briefly describe how implantation occurs.

14.    After implantation, the portion of the endometrium that overlies the developing ovum is called
    a.    decidua basalis.
    b.    decidua capsularis.
    c.    decidua luteum.
    d.    decidua vera.

15.    The mesoderm germ layer gives rise to the following structures:
    a.    Alimentary canal, lungs, liver, and bladder
    b.    Circulatory system, skin epithelium, and reproductive organs
    c.    Muscles, lungs, and circulatory system
    d.    Nervous system, lungs, and genitourinary system

## Embryonic Membranes/Amniotic Fluid

16.    The embryonic membranes begin to form at the time of implantation. Two distinct membranes

    develop, the (a) _____ and the (b) _____.

17.    Describe the normal amount and composition of amniotic fluid.

18.    Using the terms from question 14 and your answers to question 16, fill in the blanks on
    Figure 4–1 on page 36, describing the early development of the baby.

19.    List four functions of amniotic fluid.

    a.

    b.

    c.

    d.

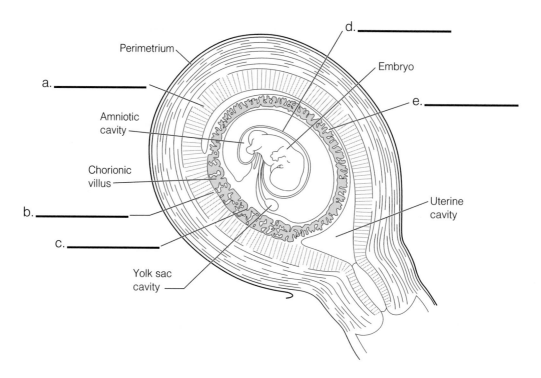

**Figure 4–1**    Early development of the baby. This figure depicts early development of selected structures at approximately 8 weeks.

## Placenta Development and Function

20.    Briefly describe the process through which the placenta and its component structures develop. Also describe the appearance of the maternal and fetal side of the placenta.

21.    Identify three major functions of the placenta.

a.

b.

c.

22.    List the four major placental hormones and their function during pregnancy.

| Hormone | Function |
| --- | --- |
| a. | |
| b. | |
| c. | |
| d. | |

23.    Describe the visual assessments you would want to make of the placenta after birth.

24.    Describe the following stages of human development in utero.

    a.    Embryo

    b.    Fetus

## Fetal Circulation

25. The body stalk, which attaches the embryo to the yolk sac, will develop into the umbilical cord. The umbilical cord is made up of (a) _____ vein(s), (b) _____ artery(ies), and specialized connective tissue called (c) _____, whose function is to (d) _____ _____.

26. Label the following structures in Figure 4–2 below and, **using arrows,** trace the normal pathway of fetal circulation:

Umbilical vein    Ductus arteriosus
Foramen ovale     Inferior vena cava
Ductus venosus    Umbilical arteries

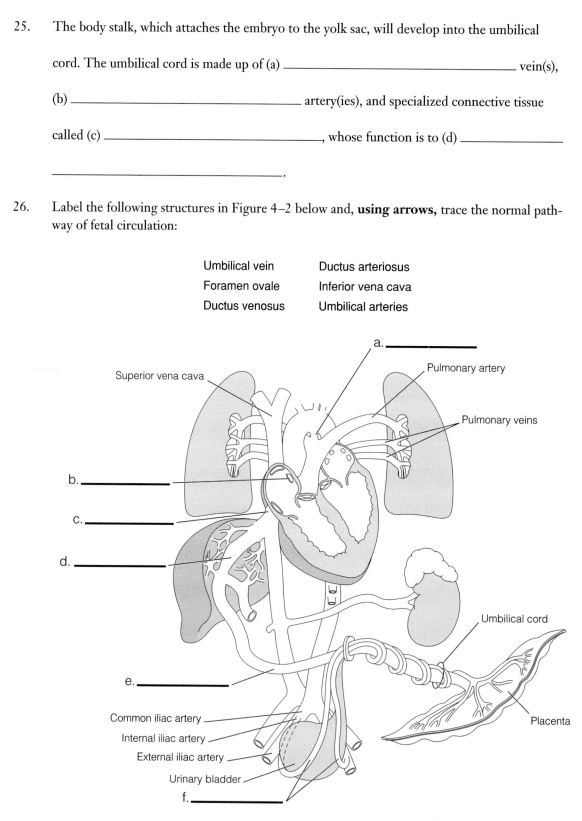

**Figure 4–2** Fetal circulation.

27.    Circle the answer that correctly completes these sentences.

The umbilical vein carries (**oxygenated**) or (**deoxygenated**) blood (**to**) or (**away from**) the fetus.

The umbilical arteries carry (**oxygenated**) or (**deoxygenated**) blood (**from**) or (**to**) the fetus to the

placenta.

28.    Describe the function of each of the following fetal structures during fetal life and the changes
that occur after birth.

| Fetal | Newborn |
|---|---|
|  |  |

a.    Umbilical vein

b.    Ductus venosus

c.    Inferior vena cava

d.    Foramen ovale

e.    Ductus arteriosus

f.    Umbilical arteries

# Fetal Development

29.   A fetus weighing about 300 g and measuring 18 cm in length who can actively suck and swallow amniotic fluid is approximately how many weeks' gestation?

   a.   14 weeks

   b.   18 weeks

   c.   20 weeks

   d.   24 weeks

30.   You are assisting in a prenatal class on fetal development. Mrs. Elizabeth Oliver, a 22-year-old primigravida, is 14 weeks' pregnant and has the following questions. Based on your knowledge of fetal development, how would you respond?

   a.   "When will my baby look like a baby?"

   b.   "How long is my baby now and how much does it weigh?"

   c.   "When will I feel my baby move?"

   d.   "When will my baby's heart start beating?"

   e.   "When can my baby's sex be identified?"

   f.   "Can my baby open its eyes?"

31.   Identify four factors that influence embryonic and fetal development.

   a.

   b.

   c.

   d.

## REFLECTIONS

Feeling movement brings images of the future baby to moms and dads. What have parents told you about this, or what have you personally felt?

_____

_____

_____

_____

_____

_____

_____

_____

_____

_____

32.     The fetus is most vulnerable to congenital malformation development during the first

        _____ weeks of life.

## Infertility

33.     Define the following terms:

        a.   Primary infertility

        b.   Secondary infertility

34.   During a routine annual examination, your client tells you that she and her husband have been trying to conceive a child for about eight months but have been unsuccessful. She asks you if there are any actions they can take to increase her chances of getting pregnant. What information would you give her?

35.   Describe the correct procedure for taking the basal body temperature (BBT) and the changes in BBT that will occur throughout a woman's cycle if she is ovulating.

Match the tests below with their correct procedure or purpose.

36.   _____   Cervical mucus tests (ferning, spinnbarkeit)

a.   Detects changes in cervical mucus due to changing estrogen levels

37.   _____   Endometrial biopsy

b.   Examines uterine cavity and tubes using contrast media instilled through the cervix

38.   _____   Postcoital examination (Huhner Test)

c.   Examines cervical mucus for sperm motility

39.   _____   Hysterosalpingography

d.   Examines uterine lining for secretory changes and receptivity to implantation

40.   _____   Gonadotropin levels (LH, FSH assays)

e.   Detects ovulation and corpus luteum function

41.   _____   Progesterone assay

f.   Determines sperm and cervical mucus compatibility and interaction with this immunological test

42.   _____   Sperm immobilization antigen antibody test

g.   Detects follicular development and ovulatory function

43.    Discuss semen analysis as a diagnostic tool in an infertility workup. How is the semen collected? What findings indicate a normal semen analysis?

A sperm count below ——————— million/mL indicates probable infertility.

44.    For each of the following medications used to treat infertility, summarize the purpose, method of administration, and possible side effects:

a.    Clomiphene citrate (Clomid, Serophene)

b.    Human menopausal gonadotropin (Pergonal)

c.    Bromocriptine (Parlodel)

d.    Gonadotropin-releasing hormone (GnRH)

45. Victor Priolo's father has Huntington's disease, and Victor is exhibiting mild symptoms of the disorder. In order to eliminate any possibility of transmitting the disease to their offspring, Victor and his wife, Ann, are considering artificial insemination. An effective procedure would be to use

   a. donor sperm, implanted in Ann.

   b. Victor's sperm, implanted in a surrogate mother.

   c. Victor's sperm, implanted in Ann after genetic restructuring.

   d. donor sperm, implanted in Victor's sterilized testes.

46. Briefly describe the following reproductive technologies:

   a. Artificial insemination

   b. In vitro fertilization (IVF)

   c. Gamete intrafallopian transfer (GIFT)

   d. Zygote intrafallopian transfer (ZIFT)

   e. Micromanipulation and blastomere analysis

47. As a nurse working in an office that focuses on infertility evaluation and treatment, it is your responsibility to coordinate care for couples, provide ongoing information and teaching, and evaluate the couple's psychosocial status. Dorothy O'Connor, age 37, has had extensive testing and treatment in an effort to correct her infertility, but all approaches have failed. During a conversation with you, Dorothy expresses the feeling that she is a failure as a woman and a wife. She states, "We both think that children are an important part of marriage, but because of me, because my body can't do what it should, we are the losers. I am such a failure as a woman." Based on this information, formulate a possible nursing diagnosis that might apply.

48.    Identify some of the defining characteristics that led you to this diagnosis.

49.    For infertile couples, the most difficult aspect of their problem is likely to be the

   a.    financial burden.

   b.    emotional aspect.

   c.    painful and time-consuming testing.

   d.    decision to adopt or remain childless.

## Genetic Disorders

50.    The pictorial analysis of an individual's chromosomes is called a _____.

51.    Amy Schwartz has cystic fibrosis. Because this is a condition of autosomal recessive inheritance, the nurse knows Amy most likely inherited the disease from

   a.    her mother.

   b.    her father.

   c.    both parents, who are carriers of the abnormal gene.

   d.    neither parent, but as a result of a toxic environment in utero.

52.    Your client's husband, who was adopted as an infant, has just been diagnosed as having Huntington's chorea. Your client asks you what the possibility is that their two children will develop the disease. What is the correct answer? Diagram the pattern of inheritance, demonstrating your rationale for your response.

53.    If one parent has cystic fibrosis and the other has normal genes, what is the probability that their children will have cystic fibrosis? Diagram your rationale for your response.

54.    Identify the genetic problems that certain ethnic or age groups may be at risk for developing.

55.    Draw a family tree (pedigree) for your family as far back as your grandparents, if possible. Are there any conditions your family considers hereditary? Don't forget to include findings such as high blood pressure, obesity, and diabetes. If you are not familiar with drawing family trees (pedigrees), you may find it helpful to consult a physical assessment text.

56.    **Memory Check:** Define the following abbreviations.

a.   AF                                          d.   hCS

b.   BBT                                         e.   hMG

c.   hCG                                         f.   hPL

# Internet Resources

**http://medstat.med.utah.edu/kw/human_reprod**
The University of Utah Health Sciences Center web site contains an index of clips, slides, and case studies on human reproduction. The site offers extensive information on infertility, including video presentations.

**http://stinley.creighton.edu/isongnet/index.html**
International Society of Nurses in Genetics web site features current information on human genetics. The site also offers a forum for professional networking and discussion.

# 5 Physical and Psychologic Changes of Pregnancy

During pregnancy, a woman's body undergoes a variety of changes designed to facilitate the growth and optimal maintenance of her developing fetus. Although the changes in her reproductive tract are the most dramatic, virtually all systems of her body are affected. In addition to physical changes, major psychologic changes occur as the couple adjusts to the fact that they will soon be parents.

This topic first focuses on preparation for pregnancy and childbirth. It then addresses the physical and psychologic changes that occur in preparation for childbirth. Subsequent topics explore the nursing assessments and interventions that should accompany these changes.

This topic corresponds to Chapters 9 and 10 in the sixth edition of *Maternal-Newborn Nursing: A Family and Community-Based Approach*.

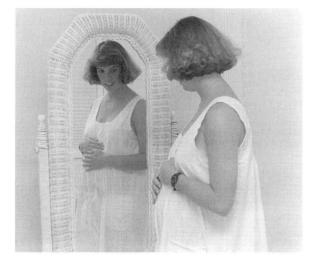

## Preparation for Pregnancy and Childbirth

1. Chloe and Max are planning to begin their family soon. Chloe asks what she should do before she becomes pregnant to help ensure a successful pregnancy. What would you tell her?

2. Define *birth plan*.

3.  During pregnancy, the expectant woman and her family begin to plan for their childbirth experience. Identify at least six issues a family should consider in their decision making.

    a.

    b.

    c.

    d.

    e.

    f.

4.  Compare the psychoprophylactic (Lamaze) method of childbirth preparation to a method commonly used in your area with regard to philosophy and basic approaches.

# Anatomy and Physiology of Pregnancy

5.  The primary cause of uterine enlargement during pregnancy is the
    a.  engorgement of preexisting vascular structures.
    b.  formation of an additional layer of uterine musculature.
    c.  hypertrophy of preexisting myometrial cells.
    d.  increased number of myometrial cells.

6.  How are the circulatory requirements of the uterus affected by pregnancy?

7.  Many of the changes that occur in the pelvic organs during pregnancy are named. For each of the following changes, identify its correct name:

    a.  The deep reddish-purple coloration of the mucosa of the cervix, vagina, and vulva is called

        _____ sign.

    b.  The softening of the cervix that occurs is called _____ sign.

    c.  The softening of the isthmus of the uterus is called _____ sign.

8.  During pregnancy, the increased number and activity of the endocervical glands are responsible for

    a.  a marked softening of the cervix.

    b.  a thinner, more watery mucosal discharge.

    c.  the development of Chadwick's sign.

    d.  the formation of the mucous plug.

9.  What function does the mucous plug serve?

10. The ovaries _____ ovum production during pregnancy.

11. During the first 10–12 weeks of pregnancy, the corpus luteum

    a.  gradually regresses and becomes obliterated.

    b.  secretes estrogen to maintain the pregnancy.

    c.  secretes human chorionic gonadotropin to maintain the pregnancy.

    d.  secretes progesterone to maintain the pregnancy.

12. What is the significance of the increased acidity of the vaginal secretions during pregnancy?

13. Describe the breast changes that occur during pregnancy with regard to the following:

    a.  Size

    b.  Pigmentation

    c.  Montgomery's tubercles

14.    Why is there an increased tendency toward nasal stuffiness and epistaxis during pregnancy?

For the components of the cardiovascular system listed below, indicate whether there is normally an increase (**I**) or a decrease (**D**) during pregnancy.

15.    _____    Blood pressure

16.    _____    Erythrocyte volume

17.    _____    Cardiac output

18.    _____    Hematocrit

19.    _____    Pulse

20.    The pseudoanemia of pregnancy is caused by

    a.    a greater increase in plasma volume than in hemoglobin levels.

    b.    decreased hemoglobin levels.

    c.    a decrease in both plasma volume and hemoglobin levels.

    d.    increased plasma volume without a comparable increase in hemoglobin levels.

21.    During pregnancy, the enlarging uterus may cause pressure on the vena cava when the woman

    lies supine, interfering with returning blood flow. As a result the woman may feel dizzy and

    clammy, and her blood pressure may decrease. This condition is called the (a) _____

    _____ syndrome, (b) _____ compression, or

    (c) _____ syndrome.

22.    Constipation during pregnancy is usually the result of

    a.    prolonged stomach emptying time and decreased intestinal motility.

    b.    increased peristalsis and flatulence.

    c.    increased cardiac workload resulting in delayed peristalsis.

    d.    reflux of acidic gastric contents and hypochlorhydria.

23.    Identify the causes of each of the following discomforts of pregnancy:

   a.   Heartburn

   b.   Hemorrhoids

   c.   Urinary frequency

24.    Which of the following changes in kidney functioning occurs during a normal pregnancy?
   a.   Blood urea nitrogen values increase
   b.   Glomerular filtration rate increases
   c.   Renal plasma flow decreases
   d.   Renal tubular reabsorption rate decreases

Many changes occur in the skin during pregnancy. Match the terms identifying these changes with their appropriate definition:

25.    _____ Chloasma              a.   Line of darker pigmentation extending from the pubis
                                              to the umbilicus in some women

26.    _____ Striae gravidarum     b.   Small, bright red, vascular elevations of the skin often
                                              found on the chest, arms, legs, and neck

27.    _____ Spider nevi           c.   The "mask of pregnancy," an irregular pigmentation
                                              commonly found on the cheeks, forehead, and nose

28.    _____ Linea nigra           d.   Wavy, irregular, reddish streaks commonly found on
                                              the abdomen, breasts, or thighs; often referred to as
                                              "stretch marks"

29.    A pregnant woman tells you that her friends tease her about her "stomach-first, waddling
       walk." She asks why she walks this way. How would you respond?

30.    Briefly describe the functions of the following hormones in pregnancy:

a.   Human chorionic gonadotropin (hCG)

b.   Estrogen

c.   Progesterone

d.   Human placental lactogen (hPL)

e.   Relaxin

31.    Briefly discuss the proposed functions of prostaglandins during pregnancy.

32.    Describe the effects of pregnancy on the following components of the endocrine system:

a.   Thyroid

b.   Pancreas

c.   Pituitary

d.   Adrenals

33.   What is the recommended weight gain for a woman of normal weight before pregnancy?

_____

34.   What is the average pattern of weight gain during each trimester of pregnancy?

a.   First trimester: _____

b.   Second trimester: _____

c.   Third trimester: _____

For each of the following signs of pregnancy, indicate with an **S**, **O**, or **D** whether the sign is subjective (presumptive), objective (probable), or diagnostic (positive).

35.   _____   Amenorrhea

36.   _____   Goodell's sign

37.   _____   Fetal heart sounds

38.   _____   Urinary frequency

39.   _____   Positive pregnancy test

40.   _____   Nausea and vomiting

41.   _____   Enlargement of the abdomen

42.   _____   Quickening

43.   _____   Palpable fetal movements

44.   _____   Braxton Hicks contractions

45.   How would you explain the differences among subjective (presumptive), objective (probable), and diagnostic (positive) signs of pregnancy to an expectant mother?

# Pregnancy Tests

46.    Briefly describe each of the following pregnancy tests:

      a.    Hemagglutination-inhibition test (Pregnosticon R)

      b.    Latex agglutination tests (Gravindex and Pregnosticon slide test)

      c.    $\beta$-subunit radioimmunoassay (RIA)

      d.    Enzyme-linked immunosorbent assay (ELISA)

      e.    Immunoradiometric assay (IRMA) (Neocept; Pregnosis)

      f.    Fluoroimmunoassay (FIA) (Opus hCG; Stratus hCG)

      g.    Radioreceptor assay (RRA) (Biocept G)

47.    Why is a positive pregnancy test *not* a positive sign of pregnancy?

48.     Over-the-counter pregnancy tests determine the presence of hCG in the woman's

   a.   blood.

   b.   saliva.

   c.   urine.

   d.   vaginal secretions.

# Psychologic Response of the Expectant Family to Pregnancy

49.     Briefly summarize behaviors that are commonly seen in each trimester as a woman adjusts
        to pregnancy.

| Trimester | Behaviors |
| --- | --- |
| First trimester | |
| Second trimester | |
| Third trimester | |

50.     Discuss the possible effects of pregnancy on a woman's body image.

# REFLECTIONS

Think of some pregnant women you have known or cared for who were at different stages of pregnancy. How did their responses to pregnancy vary? What feelings did they describe? How did their partners react? Their parents? Other children in the family?

_____

_____

_____

_____

_____

_____

_____

_____

_____

51. Rubin (1984) suggests that a pregnant woman faces four main psychologic tasks as she works to maintain her intactness and that of her family while also preparing a place for her new child. Identify and briefly summarize these tasks.

    a.

    b.

    c.

    d.

52.   As her pregnancy progresses, Alana Valdez begins to see less of the women in her Young Businesswomen's Club and spends more time with two neighbors who have young children. Which of Rubin's psychologic tasks of pregnancy is she attempting to complete?

    a.   Ensuring safe passage through pregnancy, labor, and birth

    b.   Seeking acceptance of this child by others

    c.   Seeking commitment and acceptance of self as mother to the infant

    d.   Learning to give of self on behalf of child

53.   Your close friend has just received confirmation that she is 10 weeks' pregnant. She tells you that she feels some ambivalence about being pregnant and having a child, even though the pregnancy was planned. How might you respond?

54.   Like the pregnant woman, the reactions of the expectant father to pregnancy tend to vary by trimester. For each trimester, describe the commonly occurring responses of the father.

First trimester:

Second trimester:

Third trimester:

55.    Briefly explain the concept of couvade.

56.    Monica D'Angelo is 6 months' pregnant and asks for advice about how to prepare her 3-year-old son Jared for the birth of a sibling. What suggestions might you give her?

57.    Imagine you are the head nurse in a prenatal clinic that provides care for women from a variety of ethnic backgrounds. You are responsible for orienting new nurses. Summarize three or four key points for the nurses to remember when caring for women from different cultures.

58.    **Memory Check:** Define the following abbreviations.

    a.    hCG

    b.    hPL

## Internet Resources

**http://www.birthcenters.org**
The National Association of Childbearing Centers web site furnishes information on the psychological and spiritual aspects of birthing.

# 6 Nursing Assessment and Care of the Expectant Family

The antepartal period is a time of great significance for both the expectant family and the unborn child. During this time the family must adjust to the physical and psychologic changes occurring in the mother and must also come to terms with the impact a new baby will have on their own lives and roles. For the fetus, this is a time when his or her well-being is directly related to the mother's health, personal habits, and environment.

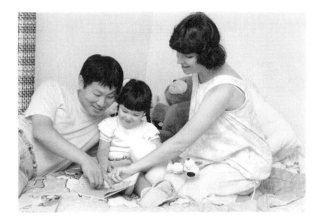

This topic is designed to assist you in identifying common antepartal changes and health needs so that you can use this knowledge in assessing antepartal families and in planning, implementing, and evaluating their care.

This topic corresponds to Chapters 11, 12, 13, and 14 in the sixth edition of *Maternal-Newborn Nursing: A Family and Community-Based Approach*.

## Prenatal Assessment

Match the terms on the left, which are used when developing a woman's obstetric history, with the definitions on the right:

1. _____ Gravida

   a. A woman who has had two or more births at more than 20 weeks' gestation

2. _____ Multipara

   b. A woman who has never been pregnant

3. _____ Nulligravida

   c. A woman who is pregnant for the first time

4. _____ Para

   d. Any pregnancy, regardless of its duration, including the present pregnancy

5. _____ Primigravida

   e. A woman who has not given birth at more than 20 weeks' gestation

   f. Birth after 20 weeks' gestation, regardless of whether the infant is born alive or dead

6.    Alexis Page is pregnant for the fourth time. She lost her first pregnancy at 12 weeks' gestation. She has two children at home. How would you record her obstetric history?

Gravida _____    Para _____    Ab _____    Living children _____

7.    a.   Yolanda Jackson is pregnant for the third time. She gave birth to a stillborn infant at 36 weeks' gestation and has a 3-year-old at home who was born at term. How would you record her obstetric history?

Gravida _____    Para _____    Ab _____    Living children _____

b.   A more detailed approach can also be used. In this approach, the meaning of *gravida* remains unchanged while *para* changes slightly to focus on the number of infants born. Use the acronym TPAL to remember *T*erm, *P*reterm, *A*bortions, *L*iving children. Using this method, how would you record Yolanda's obstetric history?

Gravida _____    Para ____   ____   ____   ____

8.    The following questionnaire is similar to many that are used when a woman initially seeks antepartal care. With a friend or family member acting as the client and you as the prenatal nurse, obtain the necessary information. (Note: This questionnaire focuses primarily on factors related to pregnancy and is not a complete history of all body systems.)

Name: _____    Age: _____    Race: _____

Address: _____    Phone: _____

Educational level: _____    Occupation: _____

Marital status: _____    Religious preference (optional): _____

Have any members of your family had the following? If so, who?

_____ Diabetes _____

_____ Cardiovascular disease _____

_____ High blood pressure _____

_____ Breast cancer _____

_____ Other types of cancer _____

_____ Multiple pregnancies _____

_____ Preeclampsia-eclampsia (pregnancy-induced hypertension) _____

_____ Congenital anomalies _____

How old were you when your menstrual periods started? _____

How often do they occur? _____

How long do they last? _____

Do you have any discomfort with your periods? _____    If so, how severe is it? _____

What is the date of the first day of your last normal menstrual period? _____

Have you had any bleeding or spotting since your last normal menstrual period? _____

Have you had any of the following diseases?

| | |
|---|---|
| _____ Chickenpox | _____ Asthma |
| _____ Mumps | _____ High blood pressure |
| _____ Three-day measles (rubella) | _____ Heart disease |
| _____ Two-week measles (rubeola) | _____ Respiratory disease |
| _____ Kidney disease | _____ Diabetes |
| _____ Frequent bladder infections | _____ Allergies |
| _____ Thyroid problems | _____ Sexually transmitted infection |
| _____ Anemia | _____ Other |

(If the woman answers *yes* to any of the above, include pertinent information in this space.)

Have you been on birth control pills? _____    If yes, when did you stop taking them? _____

Were you using any other method of contraception? _____    If so, what method? _____

How many previous pregnancies have you had? _____

Have you had any miscarriages or abortions? _____    If yes, how many? _____

How many living children do you have? _____

Have you had any stillbirths? _____    If yes, how many? _____

Gravida _____    Para _____    Ab _____

Previous children:

| | Date of birth | Sex | Birth weight | Preterm or full term |
|---|---|---|---|---|
| 1. | | | | |
| 2. | | | | |
| 3. | | | | |
| 4. | | | | |
| 5. | | | | |

Did any previous children have problems immediately after birth? _____ If yes, what occurred?

Have you had any problems with previous pregnancies? _____ If yes, what occurred?

→

*Questionnaire, continued*

Have you had any problems with previous labors and/or births? _____ If yes, what occurred?

Have you had any problems with previous postpartal periods? _____ If yes, what occurred?

Are you presently taking any prescription or nonprescription drugs? _____ If yes, please list them:

Do you smoke? _____ Number of cigarettes per day: _____

How much of the following do you drink each day? Coffee _____ Tea _____

Colas _____ Alcoholic beverages _____

What is your present weight? _____ What is your usual prepregnant weight? _____

Nursing assessment of available psychosocial data (*to be completed by nurse using information obtained from the woman or other sources*):[1]

Brief description of available support persons (include information about the father of the child such as age, occupation, involvement in the pregnancy):

Client's feelings about the pregnancy and her plans for dealing with it:

[1]This should be a brief summary of your impression of the woman, her ability to cope with her pregnancy, plans she has made, and available support systems.

Does the client have any cultural or religious practices that might influence her care or that of her child?

For the prenatal laboratory test results listed below, indicate with an **N** if the result is normal or an **A** if the result is abnormal and requires further evaluation.

9. _____ Hemoglobin 13.6 g/dL

10. _____ Hematocrit 35%

11. _____ Rubella titer 1:6

12. _____ WBC 6,200/μL

13. _____ Sickle cell screen negative

14. During the prenatal assessment, the woman is screened for risk factors. What are risk factors?

15. Give three examples of factors that increase a woman's risk during pregnancy.

a.

b.

c.

*The procedure for a complete physical examination may be reviewed in textbooks on physical assessment. This workbook focuses on those aspects of the physical examination that are directly related to assessment of the pregnancy.*

16.   Jenny Nishida, gravida 1, para 0, ab 0, is scheduled for her first obstetric examination. Identify three areas of focus in this examination.

a.

b.

c.

17.   During her examination, the nurse practitioner (or physician) measures Jenny's fundal height. How is this measured?

18.   a.   What information does fundal height provide about the pregnancy?

b.   Where would you expect to find the fundus at 12 weeks' gestation? _____

c.   At 20 weeks' gestation?_____

19.   Jenny asks you when the baby's heartbeat will be heard. When is the fetal heartbeat usually detected?

a.   With a fetoscope: _____

b.   With a Doppler: _____

20.   To complete a pelvic examination, Jenny is placed in the _____ position.

21.   Identify the three basic parts of every initial pelvic examination.

a.

b.

c.

22.   If you noted on a prenatal record that a woman had a diagonal conjugate of 9.0 cm, what possible problems might you predict for her labor?

23.   What is the purpose of Nägele's rule?

24.   How is Nägele's rule calculated?

25.   Jenny began her last normal menstrual period on March 22 of this year. Using Nägele's rule, calculate her expected date of birth (EDB).

26.   What is the recommended frequency of prenatal visits for a normal prenatal client?

27.   Identify the factors that you would consider part of your initial psychologic assessment of an antepartal family.

For each of the warning signs listed below, select a possible cause from the choices on the right. Use each answer only once.

28. _____ Dysuria              a.  Preeclampsia

29. _____ Persistent vomiting  b.  Placenta previa

30. _____ Abdominal pain       c.  Urinary tract infection

31. _____ Epigastric pain      d.  Hyperemesis gravidarum

32. _____ Vaginal bleeding     e.  Abruptio placentae

33. What would you instruct a woman to do if she experiences any of the danger signs in pregnancy?

## Common Discomforts of Pregnancy

34. From the list that follows, circle the discomforts that commonly occur during the first trimester of pregnancy:

    varicose veins, urinary frequency, nausea and vomiting,

    backache, dyspnea, flatulence, fatigue, leg cramps,

    breast tenderness, faintness, increased vaginal discharge

35. For each of the discomforts listed below, identify at least one self-care measure a pregnant woman might use to obtain relief.

    a.  Breast tenderness

    b.  Leg cramps

    c.  Nausea

d.   Constipation

e.   Backache

f.   Urinary frequency

36.   Your friend is in her early months of pregnancy and complains about morning sickness. Which of the following recommendations might you make to her?

a.   Nothing will alleviate it, and you must do your best to accept it.

b.   Eat a dry carbohydrate, such as crackers, before arising.

c.   Take large quantities of fluids with meals.

d.   Eat three meals per day and avoid eating between meals.

37.   **Critical Thinking in Practice:** The following action sequence is designed to help you think through basic clinical problems. Read the sequence below, then fill in the appropriate boxes in the flowchart on page 70.

Julie Dombrowski, gravida 1, para 0, is 12 weeks' pregnant when she comes for her second prenatal visit. She tells you that her main problem is noticeable fatigue. She states, "Sometimes I'm so tired by the end of the day that I can hardly make it home to cook supper. I can't tell you how many meals Larry has cooked lately because I don't have the energy to do it. Is something wrong with me?"

## Teaching for Self-Care During Pregnancy

38.   Mary Jo Bryant is interested in breastfeeding her baby and asks if there is anything she should do during pregnancy to prepare her breasts. What advice would you give her?

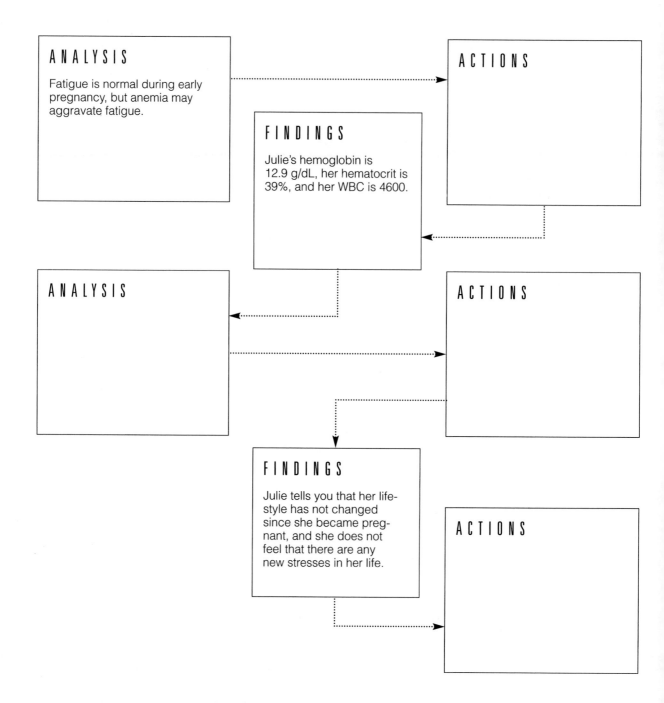

ANALYSIS

Fatigue is normal during early pregnancy, but anemia may aggravate fatigue.

ACTIONS

FINDINGS

Julie's hemoglobin is 12.9 g/dL, her hematocrit is 39%, and her WBC is 4600.

ANALYSIS

ACTIONS

FINDINGS

Julie tells you that her life-style has not changed since she became pregnant, and she does not feel that there are any new stresses in her life.

ACTIONS

39.   Mary Jo asks about the types of physical activity she can engage in during pregnancy. What guidelines would you suggest she follow when engaging in sports and physical activities?

40.    Several approaches to tracking fetal activity exist and are often referred to as a fetal movement record or fetal activity diary. Describe the procedure for tracking fetal activity that is used in your clinical facility.

41.    Linh Trang, 7 months' pregnant, asks about traveling 300 miles by car to visit her parents. Her pregnancy, to date, is normal. What advice would you give her?

42.    What advice would you give a pregnant woman who states that she is a "bath person" and prefers tub baths to showers?

43.    The pregnant woman should have a dental examination (a) _____ in her pregnancy. Dental x-rays should be (b) _____.

44.    What advice would you give a woman who is 11 weeks' pregnant and asks about having an occasional glass of wine during her pregnancy?

45.   Kathy Olsen is 7 months' pregnant with her first child. She tells you that she and her partner, Chuck, still find sexual intercourse very satisfying, although recently they have found it more comfortable to make love if Kathy assumes the superior position. Kathy says that she and Chuck recently talked about making love during the last weeks of pregnancy. They wondered if it was "okay" or if it posed a threat for Kathy or the baby. After assessing Kathy's concerns, formulate an appropriate nursing diagnosis.

46.   A substance that adversely affects the normal growth and development of the fetus is called a

_____.

## Age-Related Considerations

47.   Identify three advantages of delaying childbirth until a woman is in her 30s.

a.

b.

c.

48.   A child born to a woman over age 35 has an increased risk of

a.   cleft palate.

b.   cystic fibrosis.

c.   Down syndrome.

d.   meningomyelocele.

49.   In addition to concerns about the baby's well-being and the health of the mother, identify three concerns that many couples face when they delay childbearing until the mother is in her 30s.

a.

b.

c.

# Adolescent Pregnancy

50.    Identify at least six reasons why an adolescent might become pregnant.

a.

b.

c.

d.

e.

f.

51.    Imagine you are responsible for developing a prenatal clinic for adolescent girls. What factors about the adolescent and her development would you consider in planning your approach? Identify some specific techniques or services you would like to have available for the adolescent.

52.    For the pregnant adolescent, the most common medical complication is

a.    gestational diabetes mellitus.

b.    herpes simplex.

c.    pregnancy-induced hypertension.

d.    pyelonephritis.

## REFLECTIONS

Think about any pregnant adolescents you have cared for as a nursing student or have known. Compare their reactions to being pregnant to those of more mature pregnant women. How are they similar? Different?

_____

_____

_____

_____

_____

_____

_____

_____

53.  The goal of the National Campaign To Prevent Teen Pregnancy is to reduce the incidence of teenage pregnancy by one-third by the year 2005. Summarize some of the actions the organization has taken to achieve this goal.

# Maternal Nutrition

54. Pamela Suh, a 22-year-old primipara, who is 2 months' pregnant, is discussing nutrition with you. She is of normal weight and is very concerned about avoiding excessive weight gain. What pattern of weight gain would you recommend for her?

55. To achieve this weight gain, she should increase her daily intake by _____ kcal.

56. Which of the following menus would provide the highest amounts of protein, iron, and vitamin C?

    a.  4 oz beef, ½ c lima beans, a glass of skim milk, and ¾ c strawberries

    b.  3 oz chicken, ½ c corn, a lettuce salad, and a small banana

    c.  1 c macaroni, ¾ c peas, a glass of whole milk, and a medium pear

    d.  A scrambled egg, hashbrown potatoes, half a glass of buttermilk, and a large nectarine

For each of the vitamins or minerals listed below, select the answer that best describes its function from the column on the right.

57. _____ Vitamin A            a.  Prevents night blindness

58. _____ Vitamin E            b.  Necessary for normal blood clotting

59. _____ Vitamin K            c.  Essential to formation of connective tissue

60. _____ Vitamin C            d.  Synthesis of DNA and RNA

61. _____ Folic acid           e.  Amino acid metabolism

62. _____ Pyridoxine (B$_6$)    f.  Cellular metabolism

63. _____ Calcium              g.  Deficiency associated with neural tube defects

64. _____ Zinc                 h.  Mineralization of fetal bones and teeth

65. _____ Magnesium            i.  Antioxidation

66. Tina Ristow is a true vegetarian and will not eat any food from animal sources, including milk and eggs. What foods might she use to meet her protein and calcium requirements during pregnancy?

67. The following is a 24-hour food diary for a 26-year-old pregnant woman of normal weight. Analyze its adequacy with regard to the basic food groups.

    Breakfast:

    ¾ oz dry cereal

    ½ cup lowfat milk

    4 oz orange juice

    Lunch:

    sandwich made with 2 slices whole wheat bread, 2 oz chicken breast, lettuce, mayonnaise

    8 oz milk

    1 small chocolate bar

    Dinner:

    6 oz flounder

    tossed salad with dressing

    ½ cup rice

    1 piece of cake

    Snack:

    1½ cup vanilla ice cream

    **Analysis:**

    Dairy products:

    Meat group:

    Grains:

    Fruits and vegetables:

68.    **Memory Check:** Define the following abbreviations.

   a.   EDB


   b.   EDC


   c.   EDD


   d.   FAD


   e.   FMR


   f.   G


   g.   P


   h.   RDA

# 7 Pregnancy at Risk: Pregestational Problems

An at-risk pregnancy is one in which certain factors or groups of factors increase the possibility of morbidity or even mortality for the mother and/or fetus (or neonate). This topic focuses on preexisting conditions, such as substance abuse or maternal heart disease, that cause a pregnancy to be considered at risk.

This topic corresponds to Chapter 15 in the sixth edition of *Maternal-Newborn Nursing: A Family and Community-Based Approach*.

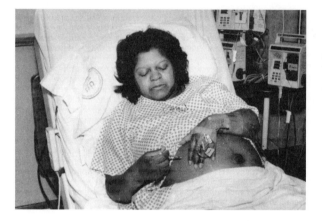

## Substance Abuse and Pregnancy

For each of the substances listed below, identify at least one possible effect on the fetus or the newborn resulting from maternal use during pregnancy:

1. Alcohol

2. Cocaine/crack

3. Heroin

4. Statistically, at least _____ out of _____ women in the United States currently is abusing a substance.

5.  Elizabeth Ivanovna, 4 months' pregnant with her first child, is seen for her first prenatal visit. During her initial history she admits that she uses cocaine regularly. As her nurse, identify at least three areas of assessment you should focus on in caring for her.

    a.

    b.

    c.

6.  What methods of pain relief are best for Elizabeth during her labor? _____
    _____

7.  True _____ or False _____: Pain medication should never be administered to a laboring

    woman who is a substance abuser. Why? _____
    _____

## Diabetes Mellitus and Pregnancy

8.  The four cardinal signs and symptoms of diabetes are

    a.  _____          c.  _____

    b.  _____          d.  _____

9.  Patrice Lewis is pregnant for the second time. Her first child weighed 9 lb, 11 oz. Her doctors perform a glucose tolerance test and discover elevated blood glucose levels. Because Patrice shows no signs of diabetes when she is not pregnant, she is best classified as having

    a.  type I diabetes mellitus.

    b.  type II diabetes mellitus.

    c.  gestational diabetes mellitus.

    d.  secondary diabetes mellitus.

10. Following birth, the infant of a woman with type I diabetes mellitus is at greatest risk for the development of

    a.  anemia.

    b.  hypercalcemia.

    c.  hyperglycemia.

    d.  hypoglycemia.

11.    Identify three ways in which pregnancy can affect diabetes.

a.

b.

c.

12.    Identify four maternal and/or fetal complications that may occur during pregnancy as a result of diabetes mellitus.

a. _____      c. _____

b. _____      d. _____

13.    **Critical Thinking Challenge:** The following situation has been included to challenge your critical thinking. Read the situation and then answer "yes" or "no" to the question below.

Belle Lee, a 29-year-old gravida 2, para 1, was diagnosed as having diabetes mellitus a year ago. Her diabetes was controlled with low doses of insulin. When her pregnancy was diagnosed at 7 weeks' gestation, her glycosylated hemoglobin was 6.4 precent and her fasting blood glucose (FBG) was 98 mg/dL. Belle missed her last two prenatal visits but states that she carefully followed her diet and insulin dosage schedule. Today's FBG is 102 mg/dL and her glycosylated hemoglobin is 7.0 percent.

**Did Belle maintain effective control?**

Yes _____         No _____

Explain your answer:

14.    You ask Belle if she can think of anything that would make it easier for her to keep her appointments. She states, "There is a satellite clinic really close to my house, but they won't see me because they say I'm high risk." You know that Belle's physician works at that clinic one day a week. You explain the situation and ask if she would be willing to see Belle there. The physician agrees, and Belle is delighted with the change. Evaluate the effectiveness of your intervention.

15.   Isadora Fleming has newly diagnosed gestational diabetes and is started on insulin in two doses, one in the morning and one before dinner. She asks why two shots are necessary. How would you respond?

16.   What advice would you give Isadora about continuing her regular exercise program?

17.   Is breastfeeding safe for women with diabetes?

      a.   yes

      b.   no

18.   A friend of yours is diagnosed as having gestational diabetes. She tells you that her grandmother takes tolbutamide (Orinase) for diabetes. Your friend asks why she can't simply take tolbutamide too. What would you tell her?

19.   Your friend also asks why infants of diabetic mothers are often large at birth. How would you explain this phenomenon?

20.   List three tests that might be performed to assess fetal status in a pregnant woman with diabetes.

      a.

      b.

      c.

21.    In broad terms, the two primary causes of anemia in pregnancy are

a.

b.

22.    Which form of anemia is the most common complication of pregnancy?

23.    Describe briefly the pathophysiology of sickle cell anemia and its potential impact on the pregnant woman and her fetus/newborn.

## HIV Infection and Pregnancy

24.    The risk of HIV infection in infants born to women who are HIV-positive is about (a) _____

percent. The prenatal use of the medication (b) _____ by HIV-positive

women helps reduce the risk of fetal transmission significantly.

25.    Identify four signs of developing complications in a pregnant HIV-positive woman.

a. _____    c. _____

b. _____    d. _____

26.    In caring for any pregnant woman, when should gloves be worn?

## REFLECTIONS

HIV/AIDS is a devastating diagnosis for childbearing women and their loved ones. How do you feel about caring for families with HIV/AIDS? Do you have any preconceived views? Take a few moments to reflect on your own beliefs and attitudes. Do they influence the care you give?

_____

_____

_____

_____

_____

_____

_____

_____

27.   According to CDC guidelines, which of the following statements about glove use is most accurate when caring for a newly born infant?

   a.   Gloves are necessary only for invasive procedures

   b    Gloves are not required

   c.   Gloves should be worn at all times

   d.   Gloves should be worn until the admission bath is done

28.   The most common method of HIV transmission for women is

   a.   heterosexual activity.

   b.   homosexual activity.

   c.   intravenous drug use.

   d.   travel to countries where HIV is endemic.

## Heart Disease and Pregnancy

29.   The New York Heart Association classification of functional capacity is used to assess the severity of cardiac disease. For each of the classes, state the expected physical activity level.

   a.   Class I


   b.   Class II


   c.   Class III


   d.   Class IV


30.   Sandy Meltzner is a 24-year-old woman who is classified as a class III cardiac client. List five signs and symptoms that would lead you to suspect cardiac decompensation in Sandy.

   a.


   b.


   c.


   d.


   e.


31.   Juanita Alvarez has a history of cardiac problems following an episode of rheumatic fever. She experiences dyspnea and palpitations when she bicycles around her neighborhood. Which classification of functional capacity best applies?
   a.   Class I
   b.   Class II
   c.   Class III
   d.   Class IV

32.   Which of the following statements about the nutritional needs of pregnant women with a cardiac condition is most accurate?

    a.   They require major increases in iron and calories but decreased sodium

    b.   They require increased protein and iron but minimized sodium intake

    c.   They require optimal amounts of all essential vitamins but restricted caloric and iron intake

    d.   They require increased iron, protein, sodium, carbohydrates, and fats

33.   Amy Chang, 10 weeks' pregnant, is seen for her first prenatal visit. She had rheumatic fever as a child and is currently classified as a class II cardiac client. In addition to iron and vitamin supplements, Amy is started on penicillin. She asks you why this was done. What would you tell her?

34.   In the absence of complications, what is the method of choice by which Amy would give birth?

35.   **Memory Check:** Define the following abbreviations.

    a.   AIDS

    b.   DM

    c.   FAS

    d.   GDM

    e.   HIV

    f.   IDDM

# Internet Resources

**http://www.noah.cuny.edu**
Substance abuse, HIV and AIDS, heart disease, and rubella are some pregnancy-at-risk factors that are examined on the New York Online Access to Health (NOAH) web site.

# 8 Pregnancy at Risk: Gestational Onset

Most pregnancies proceed without difficulty, but occasionally problems develop during a pregnancy that increase the risk for the pregnant woman and/or her fetus/neonate. This topic focuses on problems, such as bleeding or preeclampsia, which have their onset during pregnancy.

Topic 8 corresponds to Chapter 16 in the sixth edition of *Maternal-Newborn Nursing: A Family and Community-Based Approach*.

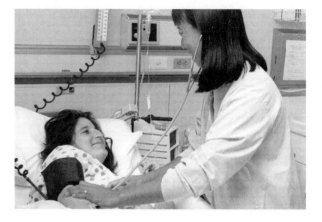

## Hyperemesis Gravidarum

1. Excessive vomiting during pregnancy is termed *hyperemesis gravidarum*. Identify the goals of therapy in treating a pregnant woman hospitalized with hyperemesis gravidarum.

# Bleeding Disorders

Match the terms below with the correct definitions:

2. _____ Threatened abortion

3. _____ Imminent abortion

4. _____ Complete abortion

5. _____ Incomplete abortion

6. _____ Missed abortion

7. _____ Habitual abortion

a. Loss of three or more successive pregnancies

b. Abortion characterized by vaginal bleeding and cramping but a closed cervical os

c. Abortion in which the fetus dies in utero but is not expelled

d. Abortion in which all the products of conception are expelled

e. Abortion characterized by bleeding, cramping, and dilatation of the cervical os

f. Abortion in which a portion of the products of conception is retained

8. Alys Roberts, a 22-year-old gravida 1, para 0, who is 11 weeks' pregnant, was admitted to the hospital with moderate vaginal bleeding and some abdominal cramping. Vaginal examination reveals that the cervix is dilated 2 cm. She is diagnosed as having an imminent abortion. Identify four nursing interventions that are indicated in caring for Alys.

a.

b.

c.

d.

9. Alys is placed on bed rest with intravenous fluids and that evening passes some of the products of conception. The following morning she has a dilation and curettage (D&C). Why is this done?

10. Alys's husband asks you why abortions occur. Identify four causes of spontaneous abortion.

    a.

    b.

    c.

    d.

11. The most common cause of second-trimester abortion is incompetent cervix. Identify two factors that may contribute to incompetent cervix.

    a.

    b.

12. A surgical procedure used to treat incompetent cervix so that a woman may successfully carry a pregnancy to term is _____.

13. Define *ectopic pregnancy*.

14. The most common implantation site in an ectopic pregnancy is the _____.

15. Ectopic pregnancy is often difficult to diagnose because its symptoms are similar to those of abdominal conditions. Identify at least five signs or symptoms of ectopic pregnancy and briefly explain why each occurs.

| Sign or Symptom | Physiologic Rationale for Occurrence |
| --- | --- |
| a. | |
| b. | |

| Sign or Symptom | Physiologic Rationale for Occurrence |
|---|---|
| c. | |
| d. | |
| e. | |

16. Which of the following signs would *not* be indicative of a ruptured tubal pregnancy?

    a. Marked lower abdominal pain

    b. Vaginal bleeding

    c. Urinary frequency

    d. Increased pulse and decreased blood pressure

17. Which of the following findings would best support a diagnosis of gestational trophoblastic disease?

    a. Elevated human chorionic gonadotropin (hCG) levels, enlarged abdomen, quickening

    b. Vaginal bleeding, absence of fetal heart tones, decreased hCG levels

    c. Visible fetal skeleton with sonography, absence of quickening, enlarged abdomen

    d. Brownish vaginal discharge, hyperemesis gravidarum, absence of fetal heart tones

18. Lisa Chan is diagnosed as having gestational trophoblastic disease. Following successful removal of the molar pregnancy, Lisa is advised to avoid pregnancy for a year and to return for periodic measurement of hCG levels. What is the rationale for this advice?

## Premature Rupture of the Membranes (PROM)

19.    Define *preterm PROM*.

20.    The most common neonatal complication of preterm PROM is _____

    _____ .

21.    The greatest risk of PROM for the pregnant woman is _____ .

22.    Fill in the following blanks: When PROM is suspected, the fluid can be tested using

    _____ . It turns _____ in the

    presence of amniotic fluid, which is more _____ (alkaline or

    acidic?) than normal vaginal secretions.

23.    Michelle Niyompong has been hospitalized for preterm PROM. Her fluid has stopped leaking
    and she is being discharged. Identify at least four issues you should address with Michelle in
    completing her discharge teaching.

    a.

    b.

    c.

    d.

## Preterm Labor

Sarah Smythe is 36 years old and is a gravida 4. She has two children at home; one was born at 35 weeks'
gestation. Sarah has also had one spontaneous abortion. She smokes 15 cigarettes a day and has an occasional
glass of wine. Sarah has a history of pyelonephritis. She has been working for the past two years in a factory.
She provides the sole financial support for the family. Her job requires that she stand in one place along a
conveyor belt and inspect parts as they pass by her. Sarah had a brief episode of vaginal bleeding at 14 weeks'
gestation, which lasted two days. Since then, the pregnancy has gone well; however, she has noted more
contractions lately.

24.    In the narrative above, circle all of Sarah's risk factors for preterm labor.

25.    Sarah asks you what she should look for this time. Identify important information to include in your answer.

26.    Sarah receives your information in a serious, thoughtful manner. At the end of your conversation, she says, "But how do I know if it's a real contraction?" What assessment techniques will you teach her?

There are many signs and symptoms associated with preterm labor. When any of the signs and symptoms of preterm labor are present, it is important for the woman to call her health care provider and be evaluated in a health care birth setting. Place an "X" beside all factors in the following list that would need further evaluation:

27.    _____  nausea

28.    _____  diarrhea

29.    _____  thirst

30.    _____  cramps in legs

31.    _____  headache (mild) relieved by resting and cool cloth to forehead

32.    _____  backache

33.    _____  unusual tiredness

34.    _____  increased appetite

35.    Sarah is admitted in preterm labor at 30 weeks' gestation and is started on intravenous magnesium sulfate ($MgSO_4$). How does this medication work to control preterm labor?

36.    The normal loading dose of $MgSO_4$ in treating preterm labor is (a) _____ g per infusion pump over 20 to 30 minutes. The maintenance dose is (b) _____ g/hr per infusion pump.

37.    The antagonist of $MgSO_4$ is _____ .

38.    When $MgSO_4$ is administered, careful nursing assessments are indicated. Identify at least five nursing assessments, the findings that would require further nursing action, and the rationale for each:

| Assessment and Findings Requiring Further Action | Rationale |
|---|---|
|  |  |
|  |  |
|  |  |
|  |  |
|  |  |

39.    **Critical Thinking Challenge:** The following situation has been included to challenge your critical thinking. Read the situation and then answer the question "yes" or "no."

a.    Helen Polawski is admitted to the birthing unit, and you will be responsible for her care. She is a gravida 4, para 3, ab 0, with 3 living children, 1 term birth, and 2 preterm births. She is at 34 weeks' gestation and is having contractions every 3 minutes of 40 seconds' duration. She states that her membranes have been ruptured since yesterday at noon (23 hours ago). In your initial assessments, you find FHR 140, T 99.2, P 92, R 18, cervical dilatation 5 cm, and Nitrazine positive.

## Is Helen candidate for treatment to stop labor?

Yes _____        No _____

Explain your answer:

40.    Ramona Aguilar is admitted in preterm labor at 32 weeks' gestation. In the first few minutes of care, many nursing actions are needed. Rank the nursing actions in order of priority. Place NA (not applicable) by those actions that could be deleted at this time.

a. _____    Apply electronic monitor to determine contraction frequency and duration and FHR

b. _____    Assess maternal B/P, TPR

c. _____    Complete all sections of the admission form

d. _____    Do a sterile vaginal examination to determine dilatation, effacement, fetal station, presentation, and position

e. _____    Use Nitrazine to test for ruptured membranes

f. _____    Weigh Ramona

g. _____    Listen to breath sounds

# Preeclampsia and Eclampsia

41. **Critical Thinking in Practice:** The following action sequence is designed to help you think through clinical problems.

You work as a professional nurse in a private obstetrician's office. Rita George, gravida 1, para 0, 37 weeks' pregnant, is in for her weekly prenatal appointment. When you weigh her you note that she has gained 2¾ lb since last week. Her pregnancy to date has been completely normal. You know that the average weight gain in the last trimester is about 1 lb/week. A large weight gain often indicates that fluid is being retained. You know that this is an early sign of preeclampsia.

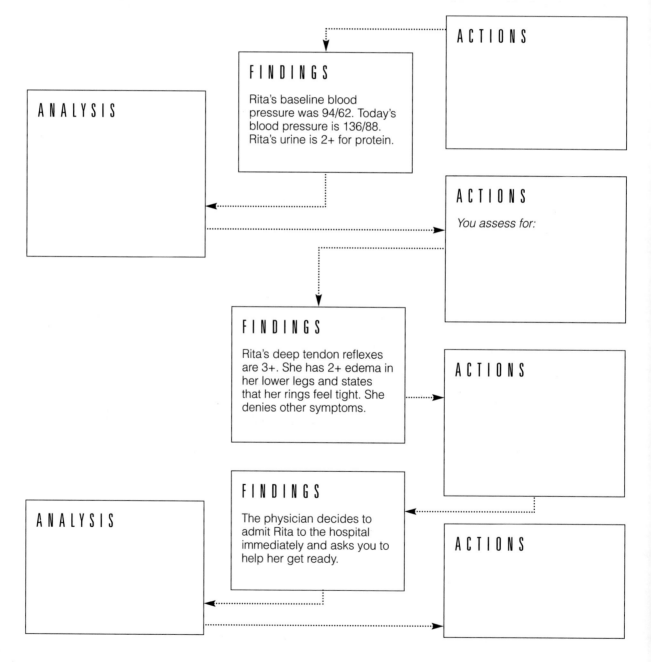

ACTIONS

FINDINGS

Rita's baseline blood pressure was 94/62. Today's blood pressure is 136/88. Rita's urine is 2+ for protein.

ANALYSIS

ACTIONS

You assess for:

FINDINGS

Rita's deep tendon reflexes are 3+. She has 2+ edema in her lower legs and states that her rings feel tight. She denies other symptoms.

ACTIONS

ANALYSIS

FINDINGS

The physician decides to admit Rita to the hospital immediately and asks you to help her get ready.

ACTIONS

ACTIONS

42.    On the following chart, compare the signs and symptoms of mild preeclampsia and severe preeclampsia (pregnancy-induced hypertension [PIH]):

| Sign | Mild Preeclampsia | Severe Preeclampsia |
|---|---|---|
| Blood pressure | | |
| Weight gain | | |
| Edema | | |
| Proteinuria | | |
| Hyperreflexia | | |
| Headache | | |
| Epigastric pain | | |
| Visual disturbances | | |

43.    What additional symptom characterizes a woman as having eclampsia rather than severe preeclampsia? _____.

44.    Women with a diagnosis of severe preeclampsia have an increased risk of

   a.    complete abortion.

   b.    placenta previa.

   c.    abruptio placentae.

   d.    none of the above.

45. Rita George is hospitalized with severe preeclampsia. Identify five interventions commonly used in caring for a woman with preeclampsia and the rationale for each.

| Intervention | Rationale |
|---|---|
| a. | |
| b. | |
| c. | |
| d. | |
| e. | |

46. You are administering intravenous magnesium sulfate to a woman with severe preeclampsia. You assess her and find her respirations are 12, her deep tendon reflexes (DTRs) are absent, and her urine output for the past 4 hours is 90 mL. What would you do?

    a. Administer calcium gluconate immediately
    b. Administer only half the dose of magnesium sulfate
    c. Continue the magnesium sulfate as ordered
    d. Stop the magnesium sulfate and notify the doctor

47. Your client, diagnosed with severe preeclampsia, is started on magnesium sulfate intravenously. In treating PIH, the normal loading dose of $MgSO_4$ is (a) _____ g given in a 20-percent solution via infusion pump over (b) _____ minutes. The maintenance dose is (c) _____ g/hour via infusion pump.

48. Three signs of magnesium toxicity are (a) _____, (b) _____, and (c) _____.

49. HELLP syndrome is a major complication of PIH. What do the letters HELLP stand for?

    H_____ E_____ L_____ L_____ P_____.

50. Deborah Hermann is admitted to the birthing center in active labor with her first pregnancy. Her blood pressure is now 140/86 (blood pressure at first prenatal visit was 110/66); she has 2+ pitting edema in her feet, ankles, and lower legs, and says that she has gained 4 lb over the last two days. You check her patellar deep tendon reflexes (DTRs). What does 3+ DTR mean?

51. As you check her DTRs, you also assess for clonus. How will you do this? What does two beats of clonus mean?

# Rh Incompatibility

52. **Critical Thinking Challenge:** The following situation has been developed to challenge your critical thinking. Read the situation and then answer the question "yes" or "no."

    Your client, Carolyn Lorenzo, a gravida 2, para 2, is Rh−; her partner is Rh+. Her first child was Rh−. She has just given birth to an Rh+ infant. Her indirect Coombs' test is positive. Her infant's direct Coombs' test is also positive.

    **Is Carolyn a candidate for Rh immune globulin (RhoGAM)?**

    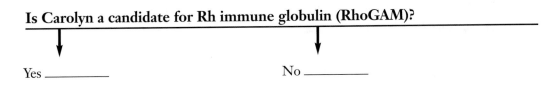

    Yes ———      No ———

    Explain your answer:

53. What does Rh immune globulin do?

54. Briefly summarize the major risks for a woman and her fetus if the woman suffers trauma from an automobile accident during pregnancy.

# Infections and Pregnancy

55. Thrush in the newborn is directly related to contact in the birth canal with which of the following organisms?

    a. *Candida albicans*

    b. *Neisseria gonorrhoeae*

    c. *Treponema pallidum*

    d. *Staphylococcus aureus*

56. In order to protect her unborn child from toxoplasmosis, a pregnant woman should

    a. avoid contact with people known to have German measles.

    b. avoid eating inadequately cooked meat.

    c. avoid sexual relations with known carriers of the causative organism.

    d. be vaccinated against it early in her pregnancy.

57. Exposure to rubella during the _____ trimester is the time of greatest risk for teratogenic effects in the fetus.

Match the maternal infections listed below with the possible implications for the fetus or the pregnancy.

58. _____ Bacterial vaginosis

    a. If untreated, newborn may develop pneumonia or conjunctivitis

59. _____ Chlamydial infection

    b. Risk of congenital infection or stillborn infant

60. _____ Gonorrhea

    c. If infection is present at time of birth, newborn may develop ophthalmia neonatorum

61. _____ Syphilis

    d. Increased risk of PROM and preterm birth

# REFLECTIONS

Think about a woman you have cared for or someone you have known whose pregnancy was considered high risk. What impact did it have on the woman and her family? How well did they cope? What actions by health care providers were helpful or not helpful?

_____

_____

_____

_____

_____

_____

_____

62.   Gretchen Houser, pregnant with her first child, has a history of genital herpes simplex virus. She tells you that she has heard that her baby can become infected by the virus and had expected to have cesarean. However, her physician has told her that it is too soon to know the method of birth. She asks you why it is too soon. How would you explain it to her?

63.    **Memory Check:** Define the following abbreviations.

a.  CID

b.  CMV

c.  DIC

d.  DTR

e.  PIH

f.  STD

g.  STI

h.  TORCH

# Assessment of Fetal Well-Being

Nurses have an important role in fetal assessment. The nurse frequently provides the one-on-one teaching regarding the purpose, procedure, and possible alternatives of each fetal test. The nurse is able to interpret test results and assist the couple in understanding the test. This topic addresses the diagnostic testing that may be done during the prenatal period.

This topic corresponds to Chapter 17 in the sixth edition of *Maternal-Newborn Nursing: A Family and Community-Based Approach*.

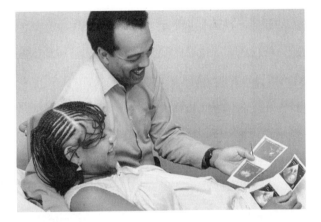

## Ultrasound

1. List two advantages for the mother and fetus of using ultrasound for assessment.

   a.

   b.

2. Identify at least six uses of ultrasound during early and late pregnancy.

| Early Pregnancy (to 24 weeks) | Late Pregnancy (over 30 weeks) |
| --- | --- |
| a. | |
| b. | |
| c. | |

| Early Pregnancy (to 24 weeks) | Late Pregnancy (over 30 weeks) |
| --- | --- |

d.

e.

f.

3.    Mrs Terrel Jackson is having an ultrasound examination. She asks, "Is it safe for my baby?" What will you say?

4.    Hazel Applegate, gravida 3, para 1, is in her 23rd week of pregnancy. Her last normal menstrual period began 5½ months ago, but she had some bleeding 4½ months ago. Your physical assessment provides the following data: The fundus is palpable at two fingerbreadths below the umbilicus; the fetal heart rate (FHR) is 140. Hazel states that she has not felt quickening. Based on this information, why do you think Hazel will have an ultrasound done?

5.    Hazel asks you what is involved in having an ultrasound. How will you respond?

## Maternal Assessment of Fetal Activity

6.    Carla Lewis is pregnant for the first time. She asks you how to monitor her baby's movements.

a.    Write out your teaching plan. On a separate sheet of paper, devise a score sheet that she could use.

b.    She asks if there is anything she can do that might affect the number of movements. How will you answer?

# Nonstress Testing

7.    What is the function of a nonstress test (NST)?

8.    Explain the procedure for performing an NST.

9.    Fetal heart rate patterns in NSTs have three classifications. Describe what a fetal monitoring strip would show in each case. What further testing may be indicated?

   a.    Reactive

   b.    Nonreactive

   c.    Unsatisfactory test

10.    What is the best test result? Why?

11.    Label each section of Figure 9–1A and B on page 104 as reactive, nonreactive, or unsatisfactory.

12.    The NST can be modified by adding a fetal acoustic stimulation test (FAST). Describe how the FAST changes the basic NST.

# Biophysical Profile

13.    A biophysical profile is completed to assess the fetus.

   a.    Discuss the specific areas assessed in this test.

   b.    How is it scored? What represents a "desirable" or "good" score?

*continued on page 105* ➡

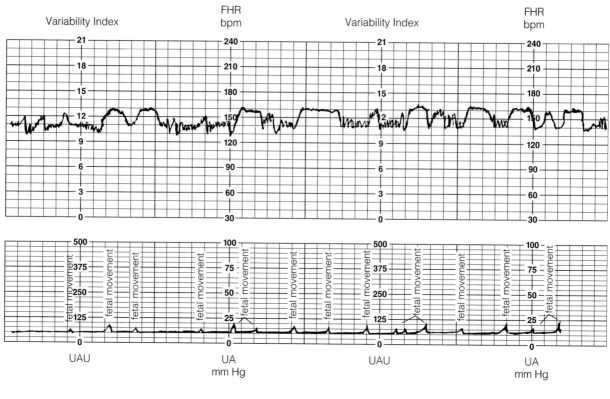

**Figure 9–1A** _____.

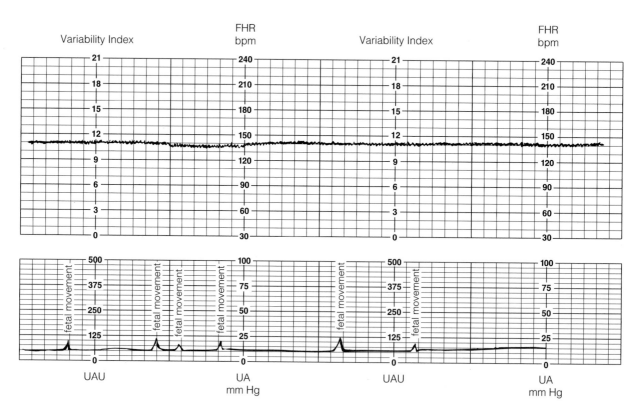

**Figure 9–1B** _____.

    c.   Describe the conditions in which it is most likely for a fetal biophysical profile to be done.

    d.   What does a decreased amniotic fluid volume mean?

    e.   Roy Kaplan calls the birth center and says, "My wife is to have a fetal biophysical profile tomorrow. What is it?" Write out how you will describe the assessment test to him.

# Contraction Stress Testing

14.    List six indications for doing a contraction stress test (CST). Describe the physiologic rationale behind each indication.

    a.

    b.

    c.

    d.

    e.

    f.

15.    List three *contraindications* for the CST. Describe the physiologic rationale behind each.

16.    Describe the procedure for the breast self-stimulation test (BSST, also called the nipple self-stimulation contraction stress test [NSCST]).

17.    Explain the major differences between BSST and CST with intravenous oxytocin (sometimes called oxytocin challenge test).

Match the CST results with their corresponding definitions.

18.    _____    Positive        a.    Late decelerations occur with 50 percent or more of the uterine contractions

19.    _____    Negative        b.    No late decelerations occur with a minimum of three uterine contractions (lasting 40–60 seconds) in a 10-minute window

20.    a.    Label the CST tracing in Figure 9–2 as positive or negative.

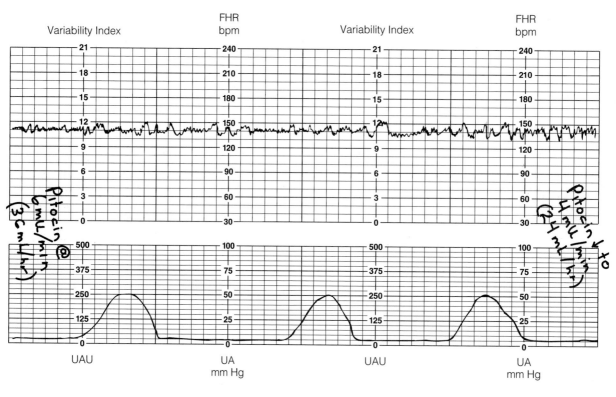

**Figure 9–2** 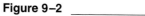.

b.    What factors led you to this conclusion?

21. On the next tracing (Figure 9–3), draw your own test results. Use different colored ink so the tracings will stand out.

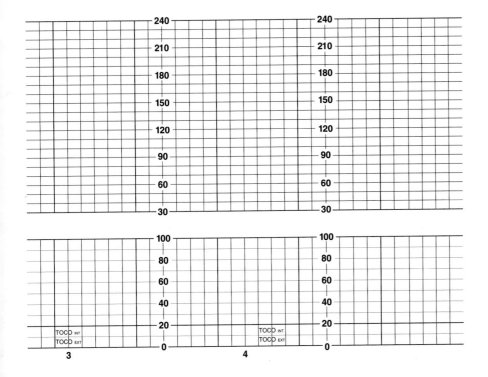

**Figure 9–3**

# Amniocentesis

22. What is the purpose of amniocentesis?

23. What method may be used to locate the placenta prior to amniocentesis?

24. List three nursing interventions necessary during amniocentesis.

    a. _____

    b. _____

    c. _____

REFLECTIONS

Talk with a pregnant woman who is having prenatal testing done. What are her needs, concerns, and fears? Does she understand the reason for the test and what the test results mean? Does she know what to expect? What advice does she have for nurses who work in the antepartal testing situation?

_____

_____

_____

_____

_____

_____

25. List three complications associated with amniocentesis and the cause of each complication.

a. _____     c. _____

b. _____

26. Complete the chart on various tests that may be performed on amniotic fluid in the later portion of pregnancy.

| Test | Purpose of Test | Normal Results | What Results Mean |
|------|-----------------|----------------|-------------------|
| Lecithin/ Sphingomyelin (L/S) Ratio | | | |
| Phosphatidylglycerol | | | |
| Creatinine | | | |

27. **Critical Thinking in Practice:** The following action sequence is designed to help you think through clinical problems.

Holly Swit, a 37-year-old primipara, had an amniocentesis today. Holly calls the antepartal testing room 5 hours after her amniocentesis and says she is having contractions. Holly is at 38 weeks' gestation.

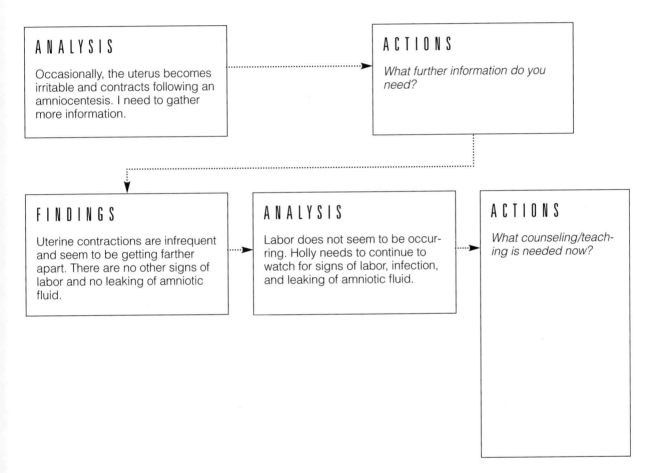

28. **Critical Thinking Challenge:** The following situation has been developed to challenge your critical thinking. Read the situation and then answer "yes" or "no" to the question on page 110.

Your client, Karen Lindblatt, is a 15-year-old gravida 1 who is in her 35th week of pregnancy. An amniocentesis is done to assess fetal lung maturity. Test results indicate an L/S ratio of 2:1 and that prostaglandin (PG) is present.

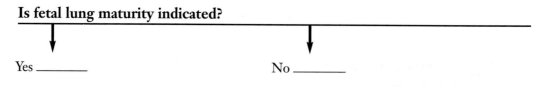

**Is fetal lung maturity indicated?**

Yes _____          No _____

Explain your answer:

29.   **Memory Check:** Define the following abbreviations.

a.   AFV                     i.   HC

b.   BSST                    j.   IUGR

c.   BPP                     k.   L/S Ratio

d.   CRL                     l.   NSCST

e.   CST                     m.   NST

f.   FAST                    n.   PG

g.   FBM                     o.   US

h.   FL                      p.   VST

# Internet Resources

**http://www.childbirth.org**
The childbirth.org web site contains a pregnancy dictionary, ultrasound photo gallery, chat room, and birth stories.

**http://home.hkstar.com/~joewoo**
Joseph Woo's Obstetric Ultrasound: A Comprehensive Guide web site describes the use of ultrasound to assess gestational age, size, and growth of the fetus.

# 10 Birth: Processes and Stages

Successful labor and birth result from the effective interplay of anatomic, physiologic, and psychologic factors. This topic considers the role of each of these factors in the process of birth. It begins with pertinent terminology and focuses on significant aspects of physiologic and psychologic changes. It then focuses on the mechanisms of labor and the stages into which labor is divided.

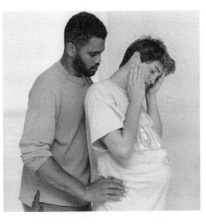

This topic corresponds to Chapter 18 in the sixth edition of *Maternal-Newborn Nursing: A Family and Community-Based Approach.*

## Maternal Pelvis

1.  The majority of women have a gynecoid pelvis. The anthropoid pelvis is the second most common pelvic type. What characteristics of these pelves make them advantageous for birth?

2.  The android and platypelloid pelves are unfavorable for vaginal birth. What unfavorable characteristics are present in each type?

3.    Draw the shape of the pelvic inlet for each type of pelvis and mark the favorable characteristics with red pen to make them stand out.

4.    The anterior-posterior diameter of the pelvic inlet is estimated from manual measurement of the

   a.    conjugate vera.

   b.    diagonal conjugate.

   c.    obstetric conjugate.

   d.    intertuberishii.

5.    The normal anterior-posterior diameter of the inlet needs to be at least

   a.    7 centimeters.

   b.    8 centimeters.

   c.    9 centimeters.

   d.    10 centimeters.

## The Fetus

6.    Label the parts of the fetal skull indicated in Figure 10–1.

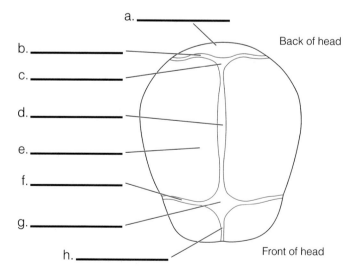

**Figure 10–1**   Superior view of the fetal skull.

7.    Define *suture.*

Match the type of suture with its location.

8.    _____ Mitotic (frontal) suture        a.    Between the parietal bones and the occipital bone

9.    _____ Sagittal suture        b.    Between the parietal bones and the frontal bones

10.    _____ Coronal suture        c.    Between the frontal bones

11.    _____ Lambdoidal suture        d.    Between the parietal bones

12.    Define *fontanelle.* Why are fontanelles important in the fetal skull?

13.    Describe the location and characteristic size of the following:

a.    Anterior fontanelle

b.    Posterior fontanelle

14.    Label the landmarks of the fetal skull indicated on Figure 10–2.

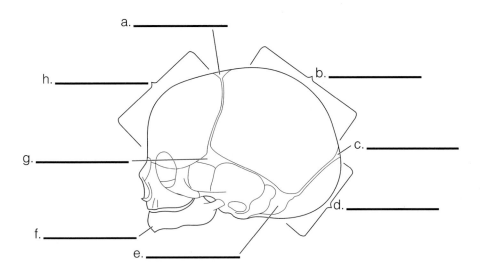

**Figure 10–2**    Lateral view of the fetal skull identifying the landmarks that have significance during birth.

15.   Figure 10–3 depicts the anteroposterior and transverse diameters of the fetal head. Label each of the diameters and state the "norms" for an average size full-term newborn.

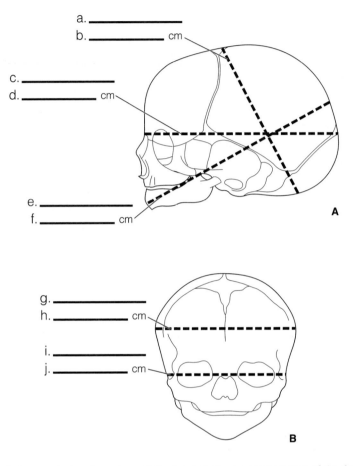

a. _____
b. _____ cm
c. _____
d. _____ cm
e. _____
f. _____ cm

g. _____
h. _____ cm
i. _____
j. _____ cm

A

B

**Figure 10–3   A.** Anteroposterior diameters of the fetal skull when the vertex of the fetus presents and the fetal head is flexed with the chin on the chest; the smallest anteroposterior diameter (suboccipitobregmatic diameter) enters the birth canal.   **B.** Transverse diameters of the fetal skull.

Match the terms below with the correct definitions.

16.   _____ Fetal attitude

a.   Relationship of the cephalocaudal axis of the fetus to the cephalocaudal axis of the woman

17.   _____ Fetal lie

b.   Relationship of the landmark on the presenting fetal part to the anterior, posterior, or sides of the maternal pelvis

18.   _____ Fetal position

c.   Relationship of the fetal parts to one another

19.     Draw a fetus in a longitudinal lie and a transverse lie on Figure 10–4.

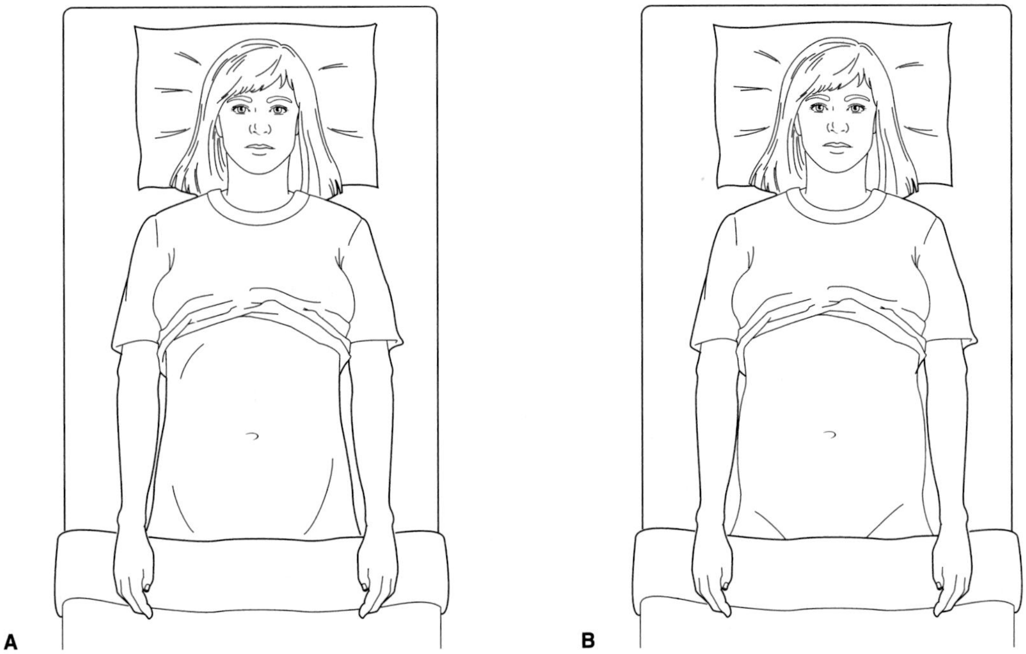

**Figure 10–4**   Fetal position.   **A.** Longitudinal lie.   **B.** Transverse lie.

20.     Define *fetal presentation*.

21.     List the four types of cephalic presentation.

a.                                          c.

b.                                          d.

22.     List and describe the three types of breech presentation. Explain how they are different.

a.

b.

c.

Label the fetal presentations and positions shown in Figure 10–5 (questions 23–35).

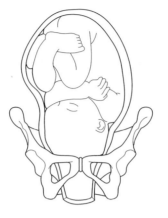

23. a. presentation _____

    b. position _____

    c. presenting part _____

24. a. presentation _____

    b. position _____

    c. presenting part _____

25. a. presentation _____

    b. position _____

    c. presenting part _____

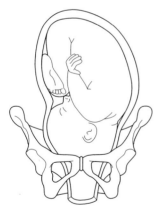
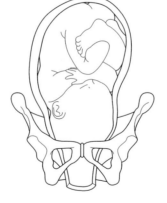
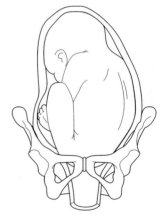

26. a. presentation _____

    b. position _____

    c. presenting part _____

27. a. presentation _____

    b. position _____

    c. presenting part _____

28. a. presentation _____

    b. position _____

    c. presenting part _____

**Figure 10–5** Categories of presentation.
*SOURCE: Courtesy Ross Laboratories, Columbus, OH.*

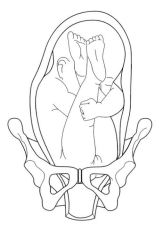

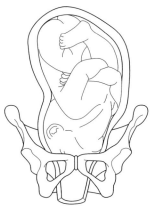

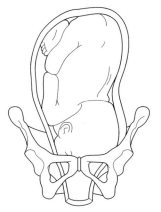

29. a. presentation _____

   b. position _____

   c. presenting part _____

30. a. presentation _____

   b. position _____

   c. presenting part _____

31. a. presentation _____

   b. position _____

   c. presenting part _____

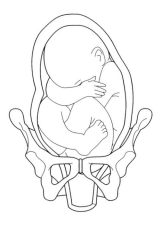

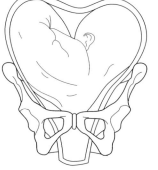

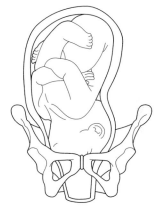

32. a. presentation _____

   b. position _____

   c. presenting part _____

33. a. presentation _____

   b. position _____

   c. presenting part _____

34. a. presentation _____

   b. position _____

   c. presenting part _____

**Figure 10–5**   Categories of presentation *(continued)*.

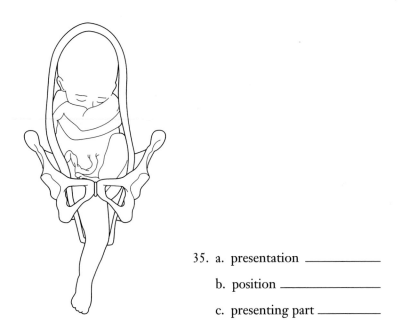

35. a. presentation _____

    b. position _____

    c. presenting part _____

**Figure 10–5** Categories of presentation *(continued).*

36. List three methods that could be used to determine presentation and position.

    a.

    b.

    c.

37. Define *engagement.*

38. What information does engagement provide about adequacy of the inlet, midpelvis, and outlet?

39. Describe two methods used to determine engagement.

    a.

    b.

56. Labor and birth are divided into four stages, each with a definite beginning and ending. Complete the following chart:

| Stage | Begins | Ends |
|---|---|---|
| First | | |
| Second | | |
| Third | | |
| Fourth | | |

57. The first stage of labor is divided into which three phases?

a.

b.

c.

**Case Study:** Read the scenario below, then answer questions 58–60 on page 122.

Joyce Visser, a primigravida, is admitted to the birthing center. Joyce states that she has been having contractions for 4 hours and her water broke just a little while ago. She is excited that she is in labor. An admission assessment reveals that the fetal heart rate is 140; the contraction frequency is every 4–5 minutes, with a duration of 40 seconds and a mild-to-moderate intensity. Her cervix is 3 cm dilated and 50-percent effaced; fetal presentation is vertex, fetal station is –2, and the Nitrazine test tape is positive for amniotic fluid.

58.    What stage and phase of labor is Joyce in?

59.    a.    How much dilatation would you expect every hour for Joyce?

       b.    How would this be different if Joyce was a multigravida?

60.    What will contractions probably be like when Joyce is in the transition phase?

---

## REFLECTIONS

Frequently the experience of labor is much different from the "norms" that textbooks address because each individual is different. What was your labor or the labor of a client like? Did it match the characteristics that you are learning about now? How was it different?

_____

_____

_____

_____

_____

_____

61.   Discuss the physiologic causes of pain during labor and birth.

62.   Identify key factors that affect the woman's response to pain.

63.   **Memory Check:** Define the following abbreviations.

a.   LADA                    l.   RMA

b.   LADP                    m.  RMP

c.   LMA                     n.   RMT

d.   LMP                     o.   ROA

e.   LMT                     p.   ROM

f.   LOA                     q.   ROP

g.   LOP                     r.   ROT

h.   LOT                     s.   RSA

i.   LSA                     t.   RSP

j.   LSP                     u.   RST

k.   LST

## Internet Resources

**http://www.hslib.washington.edu/clinical/ethnomed**
EthnoMed, a web site produced by Harborview Medical Center at the University of Washington, offers profiles of Amharic, Eritrean, Oromo, Somali, Tigrean, Cambodian, and Vietnamese cultures. Information on gender roles, religious beliefs, and pregnancy and childbirth traditions is provided.

# 11 Nursing Assessment and Care of the Intrapartal Family

The intrapartal period marks the completion of pregnancy and the beginning of a new life. It is frequently referred to as a crisis; it is certainly a time of stress, as all aspects of the laboring woman—physiologic and psychologic—are affected.

Today, the birthing nurse must have a thorough understanding of the stages and processes of labor and the ability to correlate that knowledge with observable behavior and changes in the laboring woman and those supporting her. In essence, the nurse's understanding of labor and birth forms the basis for ongoing assessment, intervention, and evaluation of care during labor and birth.

This topic emphasizes assessment, anticipated findings and their significance, and appropriate nursing interventions. Questions related to evaluation are also included to provide guidelines for determining the effectiveness of care.

This topic corresponds to Chapters 19, 20, and 21 in the sixth edition of *Maternal-Newborn Nursing: A Family and Community-Based Approach*.

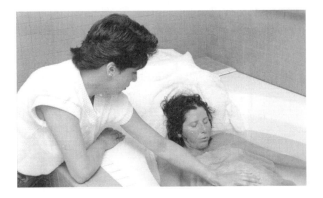

## Initial Assessment and Admission

1. The following questionnaire is similar to many that are used when a woman is admitted to the labor and birth unit. Have a friend or family member act as a client and role-play a situation in which you, as the labor and birth nurse, complete the interview. (Note: this questionnaire focuses primarily on baseline information and does not include information that would require physical assessment.)

Admission date _____ Time _____ Admitting nurse _____

Client name _____ Age _____

EDB _____ LMP _____ Length of gestation by dates _____

Attending MD/CNM _____ Pediatrician _____

Gravida _____ Para _____ Ab _____ Living children _____

Onset of labor: Spontaneous _____ Induced _____ Time _____ Bleeding _____

Membrane status: Intact _____ Ruptured _____ Time _____

→

Blood type _____ Rh _____ Serology _____ Date of serology of testing _____

Persons for maternal support during birth _____

Prenatal education classes: Yes _____ No _____ Type _____

Birthing requests: Feeding method: Breast _____ Bottle _____ Glucose water _____

Shower: Yes ___ No ___ Jacuzzi: Yes _____ No ____ Fetal monitor: Yes ___ No _____

Medication during labor: Yes _____ No _____ Regional block: Yes _____ No _____

Birth requests _____

Prepregnancy weight _____ Present weight _____ Weight gain _____

Allergy: Medications _____ Foods _____ Substances _____

Time of last food intake _____ Type _____ Fluids _____

Problems with this pregnancy _____

2.    As the woman is admitted you will also be noting other factors that can affect labor and birth.

   a.   How might the woman's culture or ethnic grouping affect the labor and birth process?

   b.   You admit a woman who is wearing a long black garment that completely covers her and a veil over her head. Her husband accompanies her. He says that no males are to enter the room. A male laboratory technician arrives to obtain a blood specimen. How will you handle this situation?

3.    Joelle LeBlanc is admitted to the birthing center accompanied by her husband, Henri. She is in early labor. During your initial interview, you discover that she is a primigravida and that her expected date of birth (EDB) is today. She has not attended prenatal classes. What four observations will you make while assessing her contractions?

   a.

   b.

   c.

   d.

4.    Why do you use your fingertips instead of the palm of your hand to palpate contractions?

5.    What would you expect Joelle's contractions to be like if she is in the latent phase?

6.    The nurse records Joelle's contractions as occurring every 5 minutes, lasting 30 seconds, and reaching mild intensity.

    a.    What is the frequency? _____

    b.    What is the duration? _____

    c.    What is the intensity? _____

7.    Henri hands you a piece of paper with a recording of contractions prior to admission. The paper shows:

| CONTRACTION BEGINS | CONTRACTION ENDS |
| --- | --- |
| 0500:00 | 0500:40 |
| 0505:00 | 0505:40 |
| 0508:00 | 0508:45 |
| 0511:00 | 0511:45 |

    a.    What is the frequency of the contractions? _____

    b.    What is the duration of the contractions? _____

8.    What differences would you perceive when palpating mild, moderate, and strong (intense) contractions?

9.    You will use a hand-held Doppler to assess fetal heart rate (FHR).

    a.    Describe the method you will use to locate the FHR.

    b.    After locating the fetal heartbeat and just before counting the FHR, you check Joelle's radial pulse. Explain the rationale for this.

    c.    How long should you listen to the FHR? At what times will it be important to assess the FHR?

10.    As part of your assessment, you perform Leopold's maneuvers on Joelle. How should she be positioned?

11.    When you do Leopold's maneuvers, you feel a firm, rounded object in the uterine fundus; a smooth surface along the right side of the uterus (mother's right side); a surface that feels more nodular on the left side of the uterus; and a body part that is rounded and even more firm just above the symphysis.

    a.    The fetal presentation is _____.

    b.    The fetal position is _____.

12.    Explain why membrane status should be ascertained before a vaginal examination is done.

13.    What effect do intact membranes have on labor progress?

14.    Explain the implications of ruptured membranes for the mother and fetus.

15.    Why do you need to know the exact time that the membranes rupture?

16.    Explain why the FHR is assessed immediately after the membranes have ruptured.

17.    Joelle says she doesn't think she wants her membranes ruptured artificially, but she's not sure. She asks, "What do you think I should do?" Write out your answer. Remember, because you want to help her be an informed consumer, your answer needs to include an assessment of Joelle's knowledge and understanding, an overview of the purpose of amniotomy, advantages, disadvantages, and any known alternatives to the amniotomy.

18.    To practice your role as client advocate, imagine you have just carefully explained an amniotomy to a woman, and she decides she doesn't want it done. The physician calls in and says, "I'm on my way to the birthing unit to see Mrs X. I'm planning to do an amniotomy if all is going well." What will your response be?

19.    While examining Mrs X, the physician says, "Hand me an amnihook so I can rupture these membranes." Mrs X quickly looks to you, shaking her head from side to side. What will you say?

20.    Joelle states that she is losing some clear fluid from her vagina when she coughs. You note that the Nitrazine test tape does not change color.

    a.    Are the membranes intact or ruptured?

    b.    What do you think the source of the clear fluid is?

21.   You do a vaginal examination on Joelle.

   a.   List the information that can be ascertained by performing a vaginal examination.

   b.   How do you position Joelle for the vaginal examination? What will you do to protect her privacy?

22.   During the vaginal examination, you find that you can place two fingers side by side in Joelle's cervix. You can feel a firm surface against the cervix and a softer triangular shape in the upper right position (between 12 and 3 on a clock). You also note a small amount of bloody show.

   a.   What is the cervical dilatation?

   b.   What is the presentation?

   c.   What is the position?

   d.   What causes the bloody show?

23.   The obstetrician has ordered a "miniprep" and a Fleet enema for Joelle if she wants them.

   a.   Joelle does not understand what a "miniprep" is. What nursing actions will you take to allow her to participate in an informed way?

   b.   What are three effects an enema may have on labor and birth?

   c.   If an enema is given, what safety factors should you consider when Joelle is ready to expel the enema?

## Breathing Techniques

24.   Choose a breathing technique commonly used in your area. Now, select a friend and teach her the breathing pattern you chose. Write a description or draw the breathing pattern so you will be ready for your clinical experience.

25.   What can you do to help Henri during the birth process? How can you assist him in supporting Joelle? Describe support and comfort measures you can teach him or that you can provide if needed.

## Fetal Monitoring

The physician has recommended fetal monitoring for a short time. After the reason for it is explained, Joelle agrees to having a monitor placed on her.

26.   Define the following terms used with fetal monitoring:

   a.   Fetal baseline

   b.   Fetal tachycardia

   c.   Fetal bradycardia

   d.   Baseline variability

   e.   Early deceleration

   f.   Late deceleration

   g.   Variable deceleration

27. Spell out the following abbreviations used in fetal monitoring:

    a. EFM

    b. FHR

    c. UA

    d. UPI

    e. HC

    f. CC

28. The normal fetal heart rate is (a) ————— to (b) ————— bpm, short-term variability is (c) —————, long-term variability is (d) ——————, there are accelerations with fetal movement, and there are (e) ————— late or variable decelerations.

29. List five possible causes of fetal tachycardia.

    a.

    b.

    c.

    d.

    e.

30. List three possible causes of fetal bradycardia.

    a.

    b.

    c.

31. List three possible causes of changes in baseline variability.

    a.

    b.

    c.

# Assessment and Support During Labor

39.    Joelle begins to indicate many signs of discomfort and anxiety. Her previous methods to increase relaxation are no longer effective. Based on your assessment, you select the nursing diagnosis *Pain* related to anxiety and difficulty maintaining relaxation. Identify at least four nursing interventions you think are important. Explain the physiologic rationale for each intervention.

   a.    **Nursing Intervention**                     **Physiologic Rationale**

   b.    Identify two anticipated outcomes or two signs that would indicate your interventions have been effective.

40.    Joelle complains of tingling and numbness in her hands and feet.

   a.    What is the cause?

   b.    List nursing interventions to assist Joelle.

   c.    Identify findings that indicate your interventions have been effective.

41.   Joelle reaches complete dilatation.

    a. Complete dilatation is _____ cm.

    b. What stage of labor is Joelle in?

42.   List signs that indicate birth is imminent.

43.   You prepare the birthing room for the birth. Describe the maternal positions that may be used during labor and birth. Identify the advantages and disadvantages of each and determine one situation in which you might suggest the use of that particular position.

44.   How often will you assess blood pressure and FHR in the second stage?

45.   Explain the support and comfort measures you or Henri can use to help Joelle feel more comfortable as birth approaches.

# Episiotomy

46.   The physician tells Joelle that an episiotomy is needed. Describe indications for an episiotomy.

47.   In Figure 11–4, draw a midline, left mediolateral, and right mediolateral episiotomy.

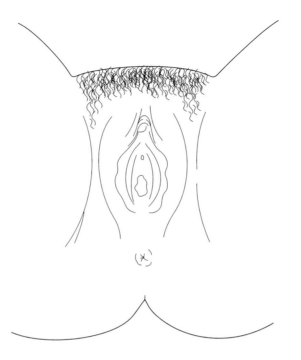

**Figure 11–4**

48.   Complete the following chart regarding differences between a midline episiotomy and medio-lateral episiotomy.

| Characteristic | Midline Episiotomy | Mediolateral Episiotomy |
| --- | --- | --- |
| Indication | | |
| Healing | | |
| Discomfort after birth | | |

49. Discuss prenatal measures and interventions during labor and birth that may decrease the need for an episiotomy.

# Birth

50. As the baby's head begins to emerge, the obstetrician/certified nurse-midwife supports it with their hand. Explain the rationale for this.

51. Why are the baby's nose and mouth suctioned as soon as the head has emerged?

# Apgar Score

52. A baby boy is born. Your first assessment of him provides the following information:
    Heart rate 124
    Respirations 24 and irregular
    Flexion and movement of all extremities
    Vigorous crying when suctioned with the bulb syringe
    Pink body with some acrocyanosis

|  | 0 | 1 | 2 |
|---|---|---|---|
| Heart rate | Absent | Slow (below 100) | Above 100 |
| Respiratory effort | Absent | Slow, irregular | Good crying |
| Muscle tone | Flaccid | Some flexion of extremities | Active motion |
| Reflex irritability | None | Grimace | Vigorous cry |
| Color | Pale, blue | Body pink, extremities blue | Completely pink |

**Figure 11–5**   Sample Apgar scoring sheet modified from Apgar V: The newborn [Apgar] scoring system: Reflection and advice. *Pediatr Clin N Am* [Aug] 1966; 13:645.

a.    Record the preceding assessments on the Apgar scoring sheet (Figure 11–5).

b.    What is the total Apgar score? _____

c.    Apgar scores are assessed at _____ minute and _____ minutes following birth.

53.    The most crucial of the Apgar assessments are the heart rate and respiration. If the baby has a pink body, what do you know about the baby's heartbeat and respiration?

# Nursing Care Following Birth

54.    List the methods that may be used to provide warmth to the newborn in the birthing room.

55.    Why should the newborn be dried thoroughly as soon after birth as possible?

56.    Joelle places her newborn on her chest with skin-to-skin contact to maintain warmth. In some birth settings the newborn may be placed under a radiant heater. Explain how the radiant heater works.

57.    As the nurse, you assess the number of vessels on the umbilical cord.

a.    Why is this important?

b.    How many vessels should there be?

58.    List two methods of ensuring correct identification of the newborn after birth.

     a.

     b.

59.    What positions may the baby be placed in to facilitate drainage of the respiratory tract?

60.    What complication may result from vigorous, frequent oral suctioning?

61.    List the areas that will be checked during a brief physical assessment of the newborn in the first few minutes after birth.

62.    Describe ways you can facilitate attachment immediately after birth.

63.    List specific maternal behaviors that would indicate Joelle is beginning to establish attachment.

# Delivery of the Placenta

64.    List four signs that indicate separation of the placenta.

   a.

   b.

   c.

   d.

65.    Describe differences between a Schultze and a Duncan expulsion of the placenta.

   a.    Method of separation from the uterine wall

   b.    Appearance of placenta at the moment of exit from the vagina

66.    Identify the complications that may be associated with a Duncan placenta.

67.    List three assessments of the expelled placenta that need to be made.

# Nursing Care in the Third Stage

68.    The obstetrician orders 10 units of Pitocin given IVP after expulsion of the placenta.

   a.    Explain the rationale for administration of an oxytocic medication following expulsion of the placenta.

   b.    Identify the most important nursing interventions when administering Pitocin.

69.   You need to record the length of each stage on Joelle's birth record, based on the following information:

     Contractions began at 0800
     Complete dilatation occurred at 1600
     Male infant delivered at 1710
     Placenta delivered at 1725

   a. First stage      _____

   b. Second stage    _____

   c. Third stage     _____

   d. Fourth stage    _____

70.   How does the length of each of Joelle's stages compare with "norms" for primigravidas?

## Nursing Care in the Fourth Stage

Joelle begins her recovery period after birth. For each of the critical nursing assessments listed, indicate the expected normal findings. Circle the correct answer.

71.   Blood pressure and pulse

   a.   same as in labor

   b.   elevated

   c.   at prepregnant level

72.   Uterine fundus height

   a.   above umbilicus

   b.   at umbilicus

   c.   below umbilicus

73. Uterine fundus—position
    a. midline
    b. to maternal right
    c. to maternal left

74. Uterine fundus—consistency
    a. firm
    b. soft
    c. not able to locate

75. Lochia—amount
    a. scant
    b. moderate
    c. heavy

76. Lochia—color
    a. rubra
    b. serosa
    c. alba

77. Lochia—presence of clots
    a. none
    b. golf ball size
    c. baseball size

78. Perineum—episiotomy
    a. suture intact
    b. some gaping of sutures

79. Perineum—bruising
    a. none to minimal
    b. marked ecchymosis

80. Perineal—swelling
    a. none or slight
    b. marked

81. Bladder distention
    a. nondistended
    b. distended

82.    What is the significance of a boggy uterus? Describe the immediate action you would take if the uterus were boggy.

83.    Joelle complains of episiotomy discomfort. List some measures that may alleviate her discomfort.

84.    The recovery period usually extends for 1–2 hours after birth. List criteria that suggest normal recovery and that indicate that frequent assessments may cease.

## Pain During Labor: Contributing Factors, Support, Analgesics, and Anesthetics

85.    List the physiologic factors that contribute to discomfort in each stage of labor.

   a.   First stage

   b.   Second stage

   c.   Third stage

86.    How do each of the following factors influence the perception of pain in the laboring woman?

a.    Cultural background

b.    Fatigue

c.    Anxiety

d.    Previous experience

87.    The nurse completes pertinent assessments of the mother, the baby, and the labor prior to administering analgesics during labor. For each of the following, indicate findings that should be present prior to administration of the analgesic.

a.    Maternal assessment

b.    Fetal assessment

c.    Labor assessment

88.    Barbara Adams, gravida 1, para 0, is in the active phase of labor. Contractions are every 3 minutes, lasting 50 seconds, and reaching moderate intensity. She is 7 cm dilated, 75-percent effaced, and at 0 station. Her membranes are intact, and the FHR is 140. With each contraction, Barbara cries out and thrashes in the bed. Her restlessness continues between contractions. She repeatedly changes positions and rolls her head from side to side. Her blood pressure and pulse rate have increased. The physician has ordered Stadol 1 mg IV when needed for pain.

a.    In the above statement, circle all the findings that indicate it would be safe to administer the ordered medication. (Note: see answer to question 87 to assist you if you are having difficulty.)

b.    Identify the three most important nursing considerations regarding administration of medication.

89.   If Barbara continues to experience discomfort and needs additional pain relief, what types of regional anesthesia might be given?

   a.   In active labor:

   b.   In second stage labor:

90.   For which of the following women would administration of analgesia seem most appropriate?

   a.   3 cm, with contractions occurring every 4 to 5 minutes, lasting 30 seconds, and reaching mild intensity

   b.   5 cm, with contractions occurring every 3 minutes, lasting 50 seconds, and reaching moderate to strong intensity; FHR 140 with good variability; woman relaxing well and breathing with contractions

   c.   7 cm, with contractions occurring every 3 minutes, lasting 50 seconds, and reaching moderate to strong intensity; FHR 140 with minimal variability and occasional late deceleration

   d.   7 cm, with contractions occurring every 3 minutes, lasting 50 seconds, and reaching moderate to strong intensity; FHR 140 with good variability; woman tense and unable to relax between contractions

91.   **Critical Thinking in Practice:** The following action sequence is designed to help you think through clinical problems. Read the sequence below, then fill in the appropriate boxes in the flowchart on page 149.

   You are the nurse in the birthing area. Carolyn Morse, a 25-year-old gravida 2, para 1, has been laboring for the past 6 hours. Suddenly you hear a low groan from her room, and then Carolyn begins to shout, "The baby is coming!" You rush to her room.

92.   **Memory Check:** Define the following abbreviations.

   a.   Ab                                    g.   HC

   b.   EDB                                   h.   LMP

   c.   EFM                                   i.   Rh

   d.   Dec                                   j.   ROM

   e.   epis                                  k.   VBAC

   f.   FHR

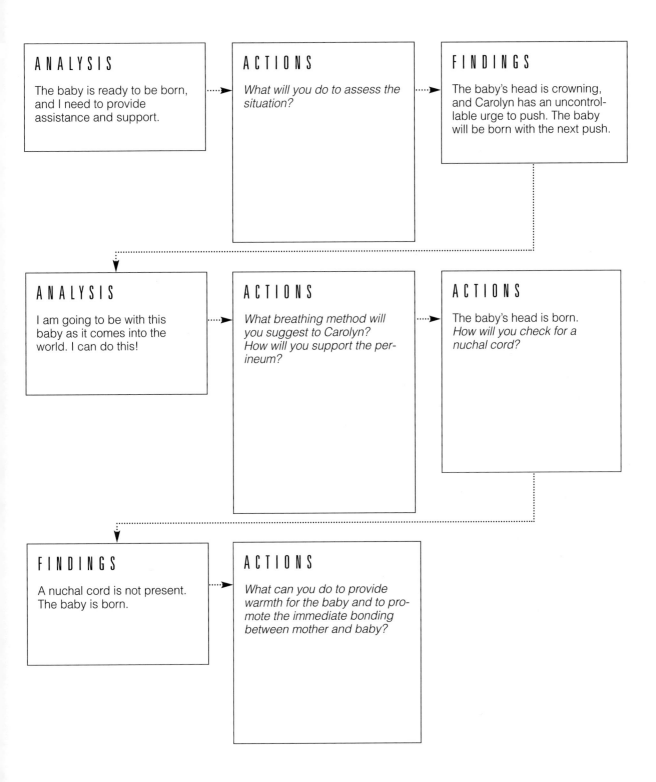

**ANALYSIS**

The baby is ready to be born, and I need to provide assistance and support.

**ACTIONS**

*What will you do to assess the situation?*

**FINDINGS**

The baby's head is crowning, and Carolyn has an uncontrollable urge to push. The baby will be born with the next push.

**ANALYSIS**

I am going to be with this baby as it comes into the world. I can do this!

**ACTIONS**

*What breathing method will you suggest to Carolyn? How will you support the perineum?*

**ACTIONS**

The baby's head is born. *How will you check for a nuchal cord?*

**FINDINGS**

A nuchal cord is not present. The baby is born.

**ACTIONS**

*What can you do to provide warmth for the baby and to promote the immediate bonding between mother and baby?*

## REFLECTIONS

Describe the first birth that you were able to attend as a student nurse. What support measures were used? Did the expectant woman have a support person? How was the newborn welcomed into the world by those present? What were your feelings?

_____

_____

_____

_____

_____

_____

_____

## Internet Resources

**http://www.rmf.org**
Risk Management Foundation of Harvard Medical Institutions web site provides clinical guidelines for obstetrical services, including procedures for record keeping and assessment and monitoring of fetal well-being.

# Childbirth at Risk

As her pregnancy advances, each woman wonders about the course of her labor and birth. Relatively smooth labor and birth of a healthy baby are, of course, the desired outcomes and are the result in the majority of cases. However, in some instances problems develop that complicate the process of birth and jeopardize the well-being of mother or baby or both. Early, accurate assessment of potential problems and appropriate therapeutic interventions are the key to achieving the best outcome possible.

This topic focuses on the complications that may arise during labor and birth. Attention is given to the etiology and clinical picture in order to assist the nurse in assessment. Implications for both mother and fetus are also presented when appropriate. Anticipated interventions are then presented. Using this knowledge the nurse will be able to evaluate the effectiveness of nursing care.

This topic corresponds to Chapters 22 and 23 in the sixth edition of *Maternal-Newborn Nursing: A Family and Community-Based Approach*.

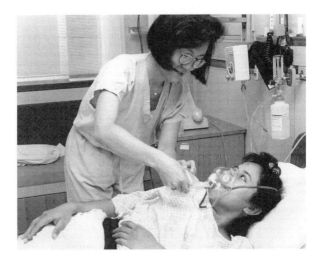

## Anxiety Regarding Labor and Birth

1.  Anxiety may have untoward effects on the laboring woman and her baby. Explain the possible effects of increased anxiety and fear on the birth process.

2.  Describe the signs and symptoms you might observe when a woman is experiencing fear and anxiety.

What nursing interventions might be helpful?

3.    As you obtain admission data you note that the male partner answers the questions. The woman avoids eye contact with you and defers to her partner. What might these dynamics suggest? If you are to engage the woman, what might you do?

## Failure to Progress

4.    Describe the type of labor contraction pattern most often present in failure to progress.

5.    Discuss the recommended treatment for failure to progress.

## Precipitous Labor and Birth

6.    Define *precipitous labor* (also called precipitate labor and birth).

7.   Discuss the medical treatment that may be suggested for subsequent births when a woman has had a precipitous labor and birth.

## Postterm Pregnancy

Laura Collins, a 21-year-old primipara, is pregnant with her first child. Laura's last menstrual period (LMP) was September 8.

8.   Her expected date of birth (EDB) is _____.

9.   On what date would her pregnancy become postterm?

10.   Laura does have a postterm pregnancy. Why will the fetus be at increased risk of having a variable deceleration pattern? What other problems may occur during labor and birth?

## Amnioinfusion

11.   Grace Yoo is also experiencing postterm pregnancy. Her CNM orders a biophysical profile to assess the fetus. The BPP is 6 with decreased amniotic fluid and a nonreactive nonstress test. The FHR exhibits numerous variable decelerations. The decision is made to treat the oligohydramnios and variable decelerations by doing an amnioinfusion and then inducing labor. What is an amnioinfusion and how do you know whether it is achieving the desired effect?

12.    What other nursing interventions might you use to assist in relieving variable decelerations?

13.    Why is the fetus at risk for meconium aspiration when oligohydramnios is present?

# Induction of Labor

14.    List two indications for induction of labor. Explain why the induction may need to be done.

   a.

   b.

15.    Patricia Gomez is scheduled for induction of labor. She is at 40 weeks' gestation. Prior to induction, a CST is obtained and the results are positive. Identify any contraindications present in the above example.

16.    List additional factors that contraindicate induction.

TABLE 12–1 Prelabor status evaluation scoring (Bishop) system

| | Assigned value | | | |
|---|---|---|---|---|
| **Factor** | **0** | **1** | **2** | **3** |
| Cervical dilatation | Closed | 1–2 cm | 3–4 cm | 5 cm or more |
| Cervical effacement | 0%–30% | 40%–50% | 60%–70% | 80% or more |
| Fetal station | –3 | –2 | –1,0 | +1 or lower |
| Cervical consistency | Firm | Moderate | Soft | |
| Cervical position | Posterior | Midposition | Anterior | |

Modified from Bishop EH: Pelvic scoring for elective induction. *Obstet Gynecol* 1964; 24:266.

17.    Explain the Bishop score (see Table 12–1). What implications would the following scores have on anticipated induction success?

    a.    Score of 3

    b.    Score of 9

18.    Amanda White is admitted for an induction. She is gravida 2, para 1, and at 42 weeks' gestation. Her membranes are intact. Amanda's obstetrician orders a continuous fetal monitor with a 15-minute baseline, followed by an intravenous induction of 10 units of Pitocin in 1000 mL of 5-percent dextrose in lactated Ringer's. The Pitocin is to be started at 1 mU/min by IV infusion pump. How many milliliters per hour will be needed to infuse 1 mU/min?

19.    Five-percent dextrose in water is not routinely used for Pitocin induction because of the risk of water intoxication. Describe the signs of water intoxication.

20.    Describe the physical assessments and the findings that indicate Amanda's infusion rate can be advanced.

21.    Identify the problems that might occur in response to the Pitocin induction.

22. After the induction has been in process for 2 hours, you palpate strong contractions and note the following information on the fetal monitoring strip (see Figure 12–1).

   a. FHR baseline is _____ bpm

   b. STV is present _____ absent _____

   c. LTV is _____

   d. Accelerations are present. Yes _____ No _____

   e. Contraction frequency is _____

   f. Contraction duration is _____

   g. Based on your assessment, should the IV Pitocin infusion rate be advanced? Explain your decision.

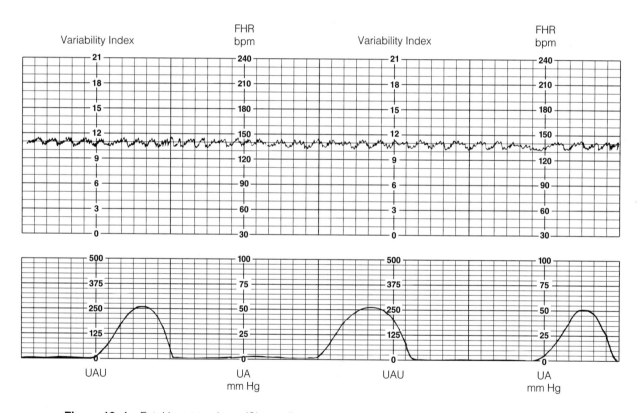

**Figure 12–1**   Fetal heart tracings. (Six small spaces equal 1 minute.)

23.    After an additional 1 hour of induction, you observe the fetal monitoring strip (see Figure 12–2). What should you do?

a.    What immediate nursing actions need to be taken?

b.    What information from the strip did you use to determine your nursing actions?

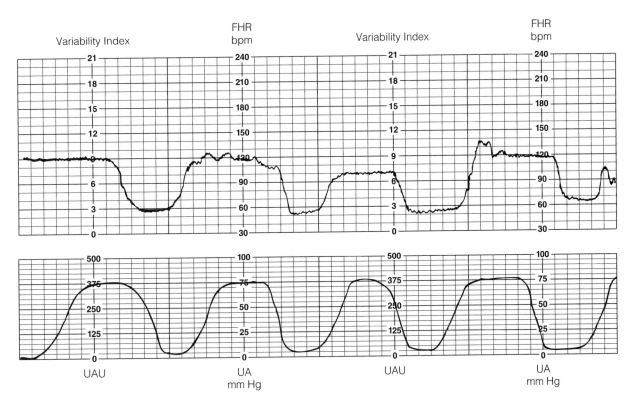

**Figure 12–2**    Fetal monitoring strip. (Six small spaces equal 1 minute.)

24. The obstetrician decides to rupture Amanda's membranes.

    a. Why might this be done?

    b. What two assessments should be made immediately after the membranes are ruptured?

25. Explain the significance of the following characteristics of amniotic fluid:

    a. Greenish color

    b. Reddish color

    c. Foul odor

26. Intravenous Pitocin may be used for augmentation of labor. Explain the differences between induction of labor and augmentation of labor.

27. Describe contraindications to augmentation.

28. If you note contraindications to the augmentation prior to beginning it, describe how you will communicate this information to the obstetrician.

# Fetal Malposition

Match the fetal malposition on the left with the descriptions on the right. More than one description may be used for each fetal malposition.

29. _____ Occiput posterior position

30. _____ Face presentation

31. _____ Brow presentation

32. _____ Transverse lie

a. Largest anteroposterior of the fetal head presents to the maternal pelvis.

b. The shoulder or acromion process is the presenting part.

c. A cesarean birth must be done.

d. The laboring woman experiences severe backache.

e. Pelvic rocking may convert the OP to OA.

f. The anteroposterior diameter of the fetal head is small, but the baby is at great risk during vaginal birth.

g. If the mentum is posterior, a cesarean is the method of birth.

33. Label each type of breech and the position of each on Figure 12–3.

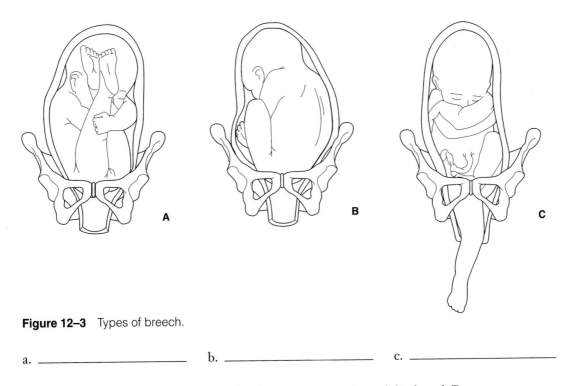

**Figure 12–3**  Types of breech.

a. _____   b. _____   c. _____

34. Breech presentation carries an increased risk of prolapse of the umbilical cord. Draw a prolapsed cord in Figure 12–3c. Use a colored pen or pencil so it will stand out.

35.    Prolapse of the cord causes pressure on the umbilical cord.

a.    Explain the fetal implications of a prolapsed cord.

b.    Describe what you would feel while performing a sterile vaginal exam and what your immediate interventions must be.

c.    On Figure 12–4, draw the type of deceleration pattern that may occur with a prolapsed cord. First draw uterine contractions with a frequency of 3 minutes.

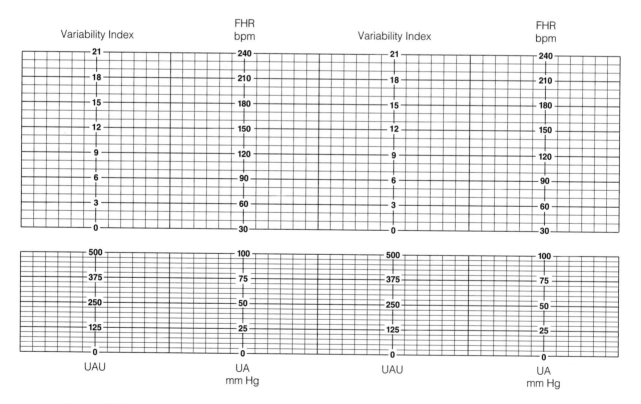

**Figure 12–4**

# External Version

36.   At 38 weeks' gestation, an external version may be done to convert a breech presentation into a cephalic presentation.

   a.   Identify the prerequisites for a version and include rationale.

   b.   Discuss nursing interventions before, during, and after the version.

   c.   Why would an Rh-negative woman need to receive RhoGAM?

   d.   Write the pertinent points you need to cover in discharge teaching.

# Multiple Pregnancy

37.   Lisa Rabotnov is in her second pregnancy. List two signs and symptoms that may indicate the presence of twins.

   a.

   b.

38.    Identify three implications of the multiple pregnancy for Lisa.

   a.

   b.

   c.

39.    Discuss the treatment that will be suggested for Lisa during her pregnancy.

40.    Discuss the implications of the multiple pregnancy for the fetuses during labor and birth.

41.    During labor, both fetuses will be monitored by electronic fetal monitoring. If one fetus begins to demonstrate problems with fetal heart rate (FHR), what will need to occur?

42.    List three signs and symptoms that would indicate fetal distress.

   a.

   b.

   c.

43.    The major maternal complication that may occur following birth of twins is (a) _____.
       This occurs because (b) _____.

# Fetal Distress: Meconium-Stained Amniotic Fluid

44.  Meleah Stone, gravida 3, para 2, is admitted with contractions occurring every 2 minutes, lasting 60 seconds, and reaching strong intensity. Her membranes ruptured spontaneously 2 hours ago, and Meleah reports the fluid has been "greenish." She is breathing well with contractions and denies any discomfort. When assessing FHR, you located it above the umbilicus, at 140 beats per minute and regular. What would you suspect?

45.  Explain the possible reasons for the presence of greenish amniotic fluid. What special measures will need to be taken for the newborn immediately after birth due to the presence of the green-stained fluid?

# Intrauterine Fetal Death

46.  Anna Marinara, a 19-year-old primipara, calls the birthing unit and tells you she hasn't felt her baby move for two days.

     a.  When she arrives, you admit her and listen for the FHR. You don't hear anything with the ultrasound Doppler. She says, "Did you hear my baby? Is she alive?" What will you say?

     b.  How would you feel in this situation?

47.  Describe nursing care that will be important for Anna and her partner.

## Placental Problems

48.   Define *abruptio placentae*. What are the different types?

49.   Define *placenta previa*. What are the different types?

Match the placental problems on the left with the descriptions on the right. Descriptions may be used more than once.

50.   _____ Abruptio placentae (marginal)     a.   Bright red bleeding without pain

51.   _____ Abruptio placentae (central)      b.   Dark red bleeding, may be associated with pain

52.   _____ Placenta previa (complete)        c.   Uterine tenderness and irritability

   d.   Normal uterine tone

   e.   Increased resting tone between contractions

   f.   Increased risk of DIC

53.   Maria Rivas-Martinez is admitted at 38 weeks' gestation with abruptio placentae. She is at increased risk for DIC and HELLP. Why are these complications more likely to develop?

54.   Dorothy Haney, gravida 3, para 1, is admitted with moderate vaginal bleeding. She is at 39 weeks' gestation. She states that she is not having contractions but that she has had episodes of vaginal bleeding since the 20th week. An ultrasound reading demonstrated a marginal placenta previa. The FHR is 140. You know that a vaginal examination is usually done on admission to assess cervical dilatation. Will you do a vaginal examination now? Give the rationale for your answer.

# Amniotic Fluid Embolism

55.    Mrs Chew is a 28-year-old gravida 2, para 1, in active labor. She suddenly begins exhibiting signs and symptoms of amniotic fluid embolus. What will you be seeing?

   a.    You know that amniotic fluid embolus is more likely in particular situations. Write a possible history for Mrs Chew that includes factors associated with amniotic fluid embolism.

   b.    Describe the medical treatment that must be initiated immediately for Mrs Chew.

# Hydramnios

56.    Hydramnios occurs when there is more than _____ mL of amniotic fluid in the uterus.

57.    Polly Buel is diagnosed as having hydramnios. List three physical changes this may cause and identify at least two self-care measures you could suggest.

58.    Identify three fetal problems associated with hydramnios and a method of identifying each problem.

   a.

   b.

   c.

59. When Polly's membranes rupture, she will be at increased risk for abruptio placentae. Explain the reason for this.

# Oligohydramnios

60. Define *oligohydramnios.*

61. Which fetal deceleration pattern are you more likely to see with oligohydramnios? Why?

62. Explain why oligohydramnios may be present when the fetus has a malformation or malfunction of the genitourinary system.

# Cephalopelvic Disproportion

63. Mrs Gonzales has a diagonal conjugate of 10 cm and converging side walls, and the fetal biparietal diameter (BPD) is 10 cm. What implications does this have for her labor and birth?

64. What types of evaluation methods would you expect to be done when cephalopelvic disproportion (CPD) is suspected?

65.    Explain the rationale for a "trial of labor" (TOL) for a woman with borderline pelvic measurements.

66.    What progress would you expect in cervical dilatation if the dilatation pattern remained within normal limits?

67.    What progress would you expect in fetal descent?

68.    In what instances would a cesarean need to be done?

69.    Give an example in which the woman might need a cesarean for one birth and not for subsequent ones.

## Forceps-Assisted Birth

70.    List three indications for the use of forceps to assist in vaginal birth.

a.

b.

c.

71.    Identify the criteria that should be met in order for the obstetrician to use forceps safely.

72.     Define the following:

    a.   Outlet forceps

    b.   Low forceps

    c.   Midforceps

73.     Identify complications (maternal and fetal) that may be associated with forceps.

74.     Discuss the nursing interventions that are necessary during an outlet forceps–assisted birth. Include the teaching that should be done.

75.     The new parents you worked with last evening during a forceps-assisted birth stop you in the hall today and ask why their baby's face is bruised and swollen on one side. They ask if it will go away. What will you tell them?

# Vacuum Extractor–Assisted Birth

76.     A vacuum extractor may be used instead of forceps.

    a.   Explain how this works.

b. Why might the baby have a "chignon"? List the important points to include in your parent teaching if the baby has a "chignon."

c. Describe the teaching that will be needed prior to the use of the vacuum extractor (include maternal and fetal information).

# Cesarean Birth

77. Janel Tadros, a 24-year-old gravida 2, para 1, at 30 weeks' gestation, is admitted to the birthing area for a repeat cesarean. Her primary (first) cesarean was done as an emergency measure when she began bleeding heavily from a complete placenta previa. The L/S ratio is 2.5:1, and PG is present.

a. Describe how you will do the abdominal perineal prep.

b. Describe the procedure for inserting an indwelling bladder catheter. What special implications does the low fetal head have on the insertion process?

c. What teaching will you provide regarding the preoperative and postoperative course?

78. Janel's physician orders an IV. You insert an 18-gauge plastic cannula into the left forearm. The IV is to run at 150 cc/hr. The drop factor is 15 gtts/cc. You will set the drip rate at

_____ gtts/min.

79. Describe the location of the incision in the uterus and advantages and disadvantages of the following types of cesarean procedures.

    a. Low segment transverse

    b. Classic

80. List the advantages and disadvantages of a low segment transverse and classic uterine incision.

    a. Low segment transverse

    b. Classic

---

## REFLECTIONS

As you think about the clinical experiences you have had with childbearing women who were experiencing problems, what one woman or couple stands out in your mind? What were your feelings during that time? What type of problem was it? What was done to help? How did the situation turn out? How did the experience change you?

_____

_____

_____

_____

_____

_____

_____

81.    As a part of Janel's preoperative nursing care, you identified **_Knowledge Deficit_** related to lack of information about the postoperative course as an important nursing diagnosis. You establish the nursing goal "Provide information regarding the expected postoperative course" and select appropriate nursing interventions to accomplish this goal. Describe objective data that will show your teaching has been effective.

82.    On her second postoperative day, Janel says to you, "I know that the cesarean was necessary and there was nothing that I did wrong but . . . why do I feel like I failed somehow?" What will you say?

83.    Describe the teaching you might do to help a father feel more comfortable during a cesarean birth.

# Vaginal Birth After Cesarean (VBAC)

84.    Becky Singh asks if she could have a vaginal birth next time even though she had a cesarean with her first birth.

   a.    Which contraindications should be assessed?

   b.    If she has a VBAC next time, she will be carefully assessed for which complications?

85. **Critical Thinking Challenge:** The following situation has been included to challenge your critical thinking. Read the situation and then select one answer.

Carla Jordano, a 22-year-old gravida 2, para 1, had a cesarean birth last time. She has a vertical incision on her abdomen and asks, "Does this mean that I can have a VBAC next time?"

**Can Carla have a VBAC with her next birth?**

Yes _____     Insufficient Data _____     No _____

Explain your answer:

86. **Memory Check:** Define the following abbreviations.

a. AROM

b. BPD

c. CPD

d. CS

e. DIC

f. ELF

g. HELLP

h. IUFD

i. mec st

j. Pit

k. TOL

l. VBAC

# Internet Resources

**http://www.birthcenters.org**
The National Association of Childbearing Centers web site offers information on birth centers, epidural analgesia and anethesia, and external breech version.

# TOPIC
# 13 Newborn Physiologic Adaptation, Assessment, Needs, and Care

The physiologic changes that occur during extrauterine adaptation are at once dramatic and yet subtle, requiring careful and continuous monitoring. Today's neonatal nurse assesses neonatal development, identifies common variations in each newborn, and recognizes abnormalities. The nurse identifies necessary early nursing interventions, initial daily care needs including breast and bottle feeding, and the discharge teaching required for successful transition to home for the parent-infant unit.

Parent teaching, a second major area of nursing responsibility, involves helping the family learn to care for its newest member.

This topic corresponds to Chapters 24, 25, 26, and 27 in the sixth edition of *Maternal-Newborn Nursing: A Family and Community-Based Approach*.

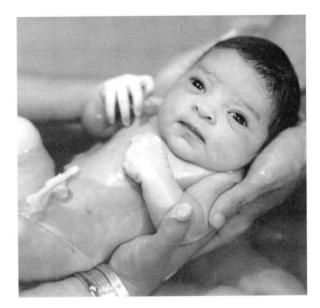

## Physiologic Adaptations

1.  Describe four factors that are thought to stimulate the newborn to take its first breath.

    a.

    b.

    c.

    d.

2.    State four anatomic and physiologic changes that occur in the cardiovascular system during
the transition from fetal to neonatal circulation.

a.

b.

c.

d.

3.    Newborn Zoe's temperature drops when she is placed on the cool plastic surface of the weight scales. This is an example of heat loss via

    a.    conduction.

    b.    convection.

    c.    evaporation.

    d.    radiation.

4.    What position do most newborns usually assume? Why?

5.    Describe the dialogue you would use to teach a new mother about physiologic jaundice. Include why the time of onset of the jaundice is important.

6.    Discuss the expected level of development of the following senses in the newborn:

| Sense | Assessment Method | Findings |
| --- | --- | --- |
| Hearing | | |
| Touch | | |
| Taste/sucking | | |
| Smell | | |
| Pain | | |

## REFLECTIONS

Do you remember the first time you held and cared for a newborn in your mother-baby rotation? How did you feel? What were your thoughts/impressions?

_____

_____

_____

_____

_____

_____

_____

## Period of Reactivity

7.   Which of the following behaviors are characteristic of the second period of reactivity?

   a.   Awake and alert, lasts 4–6 hours, sucks, swallows

   b.   Difficult to awaken, lasts 2–4 hours, bowel sounds present

   c.   Eyes open, lasts 30 minutes, strong sucking reflex

   d.   Face relaxed, regular and deep breaths, occasional startle

8.   A primary nursing intervention appropriate to the second period of reactivity would be to

   a.   auscultate the abdomen for the presence of bowel sounds.

   b.   encourage the mother to begin breastfeeding.

   c.   observe for excessive mucus.

   d.   place infant under a radiant warmer.

# Gestational Age Assessment

As part of the admission process, the newborn's gestational age is determined. Using Ballard's gestational-age scoring tool (Figure 13–1 on page 178), determine Pam's gestational age.

Pam's gestational physical exam yields the following assessments of her physical maturity: her skin is cracking and has a pale area; some areas have no lanugo present; the breast bud is 1–2 mm with stippled areola; the ears are formed and firm with instant recoil; plantar creases extend over the anterior two-thirds of the sole; and the labia majora completely cover the minora and the clitoris. Assessment of Pam's neuromuscular development shows posture with flexion of the arms and hips, 0° square window, 90°–100° arm recoil, popliteal angle of 110°, scarf sign with elbow at midline, and a score of 4 for the head-to-ear maneuver.

Pam's birth weight was 3202 g, her length was 49 cm, and her head circumference was 33.5 cm.

9.   Pam's score is (a) _____, which equates to a gestational age of

     (b) _____ weeks.

10.  Based on the gestational age you determined, correlate it with Pam's weight and classify her as

     LGA, AGA, or SGA. _____

     Plot Pam's length, weight, and head circumference on Figure 13–2 on page 179.

11.  What factors might influence the neonate's gestational age score?

12.  Why is it important to determine the gestational age of all newborns?

# NEWBORN MATURITY RATING & CLASSIFICATION

## ESTIMATION OF GESTATIONAL AGE BY MATURITY RATING
Symbols:  X - 1st Exam        O - 2nd Exam

### NEUROMUSCULAR MATURITY

| | −1 | 0 | 1 | 2 | 3 | 4 | 5 |
|---|---|---|---|---|---|---|---|
| Posture | | | | | | | |
| Square Window (wrist) | >90° | 90° | 60° | 45° | 30° | 0° | |
| Arm Recoil | | 180° | 140°−180° | 110°−140° | 90°−110° | <90° | |
| Popliteal Angle | 180° | 160° | 140° | 120° | 100° | 90° | <90° |
| Scarf Sign | | | | | | | |
| Heel to Ear | | | | | | | |

### PHYSICAL MATURITY

| | | | | | | | |
|---|---|---|---|---|---|---|---|
| Skin | sticky friable transparent | gelatinous red, translucent | smooth pink, visible veins | superficial peeling &/or rash, few veins | cracking pale areas rare veins | parchment deep cracking no vessels | leathery cracked wrinkled |
| Lanugo | none | sparse | abundant | thinning | bald areas | mostly bald | |
| Plantar Surface | heel-toe 40–50mm:−1 <40mm:−2 | >50mm no crease | faint red marks | anterior transverse crease only | creases ant. 2/3 | creases over entire sole | |
| Breast | imperceptible | barely perceptible | flat areola no bud | stippled areola 1–2mm bud | raised areola 3–4mm bud | full areola 5–10mm bud | |
| Eye/Ear | lids fused loosely:−1 tightly:−2 | lids open pinna flat stays folded | sl. curved pinna; soft; slow recoil | well curved pinna; soft but ready recoil | formed & firm instant recoil | thick cartilage ear stiff | |
| Genitals male | scrotum flat, smooth | scrotum empty faint rugae | testes in upper canal rare rugae | testes decending few rugae | testes down good rugae | testes pendulous deep rugae | |
| Genitals female | clitoris prominent labia flat | prominent clitoris small labia minora | prominent clitoris enlarging minora | majora & minora equally prominent | majora large minora small | majora cover clitoris & minora | |

Scoring system: Ballard JL, Khoury JC, Wedig K, Wang L, Eilers-Walsman BL,
Lipp R. New Ballard Score, expanded to include extremely premature infants
*J Pediatr, 1991*; 119:417–423.

Gestation by Dates _____ w

Birth Date _____ Hour _____ a
p

APGAR _____ 1 min _____ 5 m

### MATURITY RATING

| score | weeks |
|---|---|
| −10 | 20 |
| −5 | 22 |
| 0 | 24 |
| 5 | 26 |
| 10 | 28 |
| 15 | 30 |
| 20 | 32 |
| 25 | 34 |
| 30 | 36 |
| 35 | 38 |
| 40 | 40 |
| 45 | 42 |
| 50 | 44 |

### SCORING SECTION

| | 1st Exam = X | 2nd Exam = |
|---|---|---|
| Estimating Gest Age by Maturity Rating | _____Weeks | _____Week |
| Time of Exam | Date _____ Hour_____ am pm | Date _____ Hour_____ a p |
| Age at Exam | _____ Hours | _____ Hours |
| Signature of Examiner | _____ M.D. | _____ M. |

**Figure 13–1**    Ballard's gestational-age scoring tool.

## CLASSIFICATION OF NEWBORNS—
## BASED ON MATURITY AND INTRAUTERINE GROWTH

Symbols: X-1st Exam  O-2nd Exam

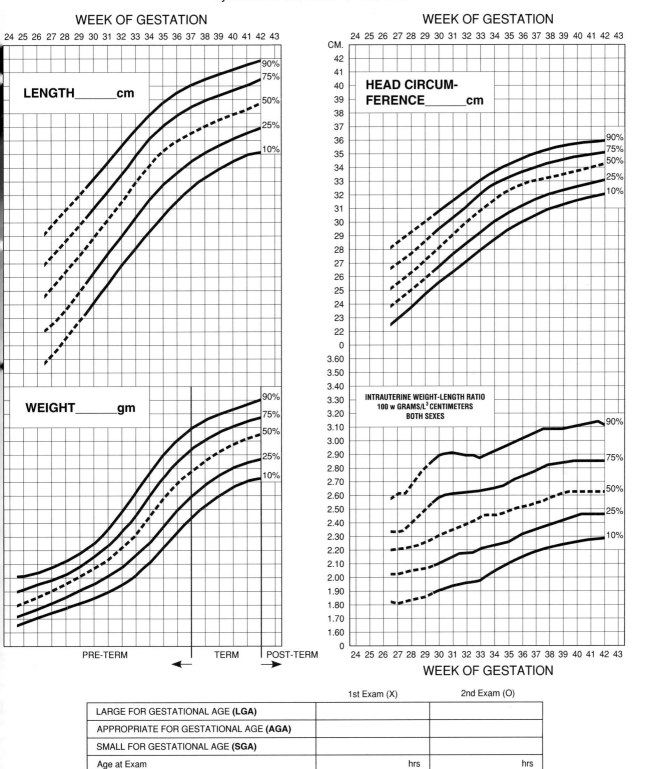

**Figure 13–2**  Intrauterine growth chart.

## Initial Assessments

13.   List the normal values for the following areas of initial assessment of the neonate:

| Assessment Area | Normal Values |
| --- | --- |
| a. Temperature | |
| b. Pulse | |
| c. Respirations | |
| d. Blood pressure | |
| e. Average weight | |
| f. Average length | |
| g. Circumference of the head | |
| h. Circumference of the chest | |

14.   Draw dotted lines on Figure 13–3 below to show where you would measure a newborn's head and chest.

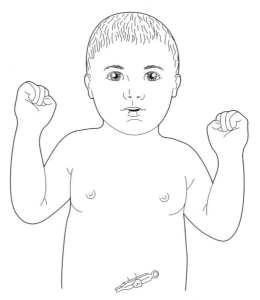

**Figure 13–3**   Measurement of newborn's head and chest.

15. Usual weight loss within the first 3–4 days of life for a full-term newborn is _____ percent.

16. Why does the newborn commonly exhibit a "physiologic weight loss"?

17. Describe how you would accurately and safely measure the newborn's length.

18. Identify each of the following newborn skin variations, differentiating them by appearance, location, and significance:

    a. Harlequin color change

    b. Erythema neonatorum toxicum

    c. Telangiectatic nevi (stork bites)

    d. Nevus flammeus (port-wine stain)

    e. Mongolian spots

    f. Nevus vasculosus (strawberry mark)

19. Which statement best defines a cephalhematoma?
    a. Diffuse edema of the scalp resulting from compression of local blood vessels
    b. Subperiosteal hemorrhage resulting from a traumatic birth
    c. Temporary reshaping of the skull resulting from the pressure of birth

20.   On Figure 13–4, draw a series of numbered circles to indicate the correct sequence for auscultating a newborn's lungs. Place an "X" at the point where you should place your stethoscope in order to count the apical pulse.

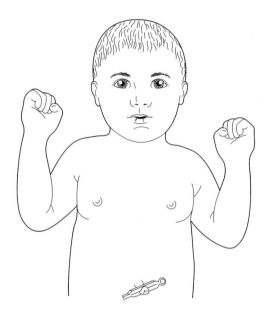

**Figure 13–4**   Auscultation of newborn's lungs and heart.

## Physical Assessment of the Newborn

21.   As the newborn nurse, you would complete an initial physical assessment of each newborn. Complete the following physical assessment chart.

| Assessment Area | Normal Findings and Common Variations |
|---|---|
| *Posture* | |
| At rest | |
| Awake | |
| *Skin* | |
| Color | |
| Pigmentation | |

| Assessment Area | Normal Findings and Common Variations |
| --- | --- |
| *Head* | |
|    Shape | |
|    Sutures | |
|    Fontanelles | |
|    Face | |
|       Eyes | |
|          Movement | |
|          Conjunctiva | |
| *Ears* | |
|    Placement | |
| *Nose* | |
|    Patency | |
| *Mouth* | |
|    Gums | |
|    Palate (hard & soft) | |
|    Tongue | |
| *Neck* | |
|    Clavicles | |

➤

| Assessment Area | Normal Findings and Common Variations |
|---|---|
| *Chest* | |
|     Shape | |
|     Point of maximal intensity (PMI) | |
|     Characteristics of pulse | |
| *Lungs* | |
|     Characteristics of breathing | |
|     Cry | |
| *Abdomen* | |
|     Umbilical cord vessels | |
| *Hips* | |
| *Extremities* | |
|     Position | |
|     Movement | |
| *Genitalia* | |
| *Spine* | |

| Assessment Area | Normal Findings and Common Variations |
|---|---|
| *Anus* <br> Placement and patency | |
| *Neuromuscular* <br> Movement and tone | |

22.    The newborn is born with various reflexes. Complete the following chart:

| Reflex | Description | How Elicited | Age at Disappearance |
|---|---|---|---|
| Moro | | | |
| Tonic neck | | | |
| Rooting | | | |
| Grasp | | | |
| Stepping | | | |
| Other | | | |

23.    Identify four protective reflexes found in all normal newborns.

a.

b.

c.

d.

24.    As you complete the newborn physical assessment, alteration in findings may be identified. Describe the defining physical characteristics or alterations, and methods of assessment used for the following:

Hydrocephalus

Facial nerve palsy

Cleft palate

Omphalocele

Hypospadias

Myelomeningocele

Congenital dislocated hip

Clubfoot

25.    Why are the newborn's hands and feet often cold?

# Care During Admission and First Four Hours of Life

You enter the birthing room to meet Ryan and his parents. Ryan is 20 minutes old and is in a quiet, alert state while interacting with his mother.

26.    What seven essential areas of information would you ascertain about Ryan's perinatal, intra-natal, and immediate postnatal period? Give your rationale.

a.

b.

c.

d.

e.

f.

g.

27.    List and prioritize eight nursing actions you would carry out during the first 4 hours (transitional period) of the newborn's life.

a.

b.

c.

d.

e.

f.

g.

h.

28.    Why is a vitamin K medication given prophylactically to newborns?

29.   **Critical Thinking in Practice:** The following action sequence is designed to help you think through basic clinical problems.

Glen, a 3450-g baby boy, is born breech to Mrs Küchler and has an Apgar score of 7 at 1 minute. Mrs Küchler has requested to breastfeed Glen on the birthing bed.

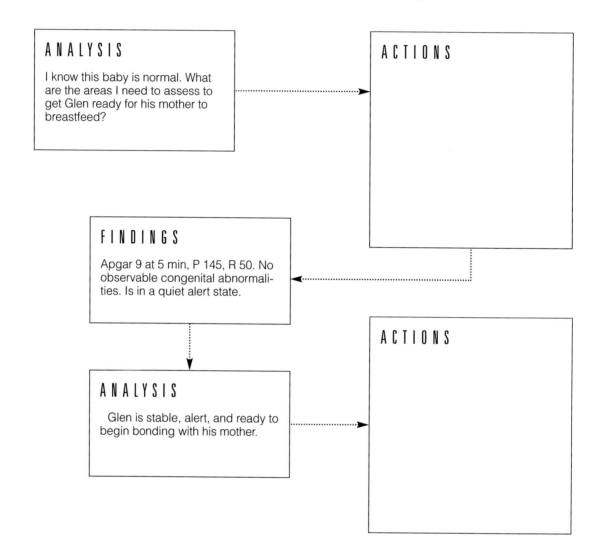

30.   What is the appropriate dosage and preferred site for administration of vitamin K?

31.   Prophylactic eye ointments are instilled in the newborn's eyes in the immediate newborn period to prevent (a) _____, which is caused by (b) _____ .

32.    List two prophylactic eye ointments that are commonly used.

a.

b.

33.    Write a sample newborn admission note.

_____

_____

_____

_____

_____

_____

_____

_____

_____

_____

At the end of the transitional period, or 4–6 hours after birth, baseline laboratory tests are completed.

34.    For each of the following laboratory values, identify the significance and appropriate nursing interventions:

| Laboratory Value | Significance | Nursing Interventions |
| --- | --- | --- |
| Central hematocrit of 68% | | |
| Hemoglobin of 12.5 g/dL | | |
| Bilirubin of 15 mg/dL | | |
| Heelstick glucose <45 mg% | | |

35.    While working in the nursery, you notice that baby Ryan, age 5 hours, has turned blue. Closer inspection reveals a large amount of frothy mucus in his mouth. What would be your nursing diagnosis in this situation? What immediate nursing interventions would you undertake?

Ryan Montoya has successfully progressed through the transitional period; he is now 6 hours old and continues to be adapting well to extrauterine life.

## Daily Newborn Nursing Assessments

36.    You are assigned to the mother-baby area. List seven daily assessments that are made of each newborn.

a.


b.


c.


d.


e.


f.


g.

37.    Write a sample of a daily newborn nursing note.

_____

_____

_____

_____

_____

_____

_____

38.    Ryan is now 12 hours old. He voids as you begin to change his diaper. What observations should you make about his voiding?

39.    If Ryan had failed to void within 24 hours after birth, describe the assessments you would carry out.

40.    Within how many hours after birth would you expect Ryan to have his first stool and what would its appearance be?

# Breastfeeding

41.    Helena Montoya wants to breastfeed Ryan. She tells you that she is really interested in breast-feeding but feels overwhelmed because she has so many questions and feels uncertain about beginning. She states, "I feel so full of questions that I wonder if I will ever know what to do." Based on your analysis of this data, formulate a nursing diagnosis that might apply.

42.    Based on your diagnosis, what information would you give Helena about breastfeeding her son?

   a.    Methods for encouraging the baby to nurse


   b.    Positions for feeding


   c.    Let-down reflex


   d.    Breaking suction before removing the infant from the breast


   e.    Length of time per breast


   f.    Frequency of feeding


43.    You stay and assist Helena with breastfeeding and answer her questions. Once she appears comfortable, you leave, but you check back with her periodically. Later in the morning when her baby is sleeping, you return to share information about other areas related to successful breastfeeding. What information would you share with Helena about the following areas?

   a.    Nipple care


   b.    Breast support


   c.    Relief measures for breast engorgement


   d.    Maternal nutrition while breastfeeding


   e.    Environmental influences on successful breastfeeding

f.   Use of medications while breastfeeding

g.   Personal support systems

h.   Available community resources

44.   Helena is scheduled to remain on postpartum for only 24–48 hours. What actions can you take to help reinforce her learning so that things will go more smoothly when she is home?

45.   How will you evaluate the effectiveness of your teaching plan in meeting Helena's education needs?

46.   How would you evaluate the adequacy of Helena's fluid and nutritional intake while being breastfed?

Christy is a 2-day-old, bottle-fed, 3175-g infant. During a follow-up call, her mother is concerned because "she takes only 1½ oz at each feeding."

47.   What would your response be?

48.   List at least five points to be included in a teaching plan to help Christy's mom successfully bottle-feed.

a.

b.



c.



d.



e.


49.    When bottle-feeding her son, the nurse observes that Mrs Paar attempts to burp him after every few swallows of formula. He becomes restless and cries, upsetting Mrs.Paar. Which response by the nurse is most appropriate?

a.    "You're burping him much too frequently, Mrs Paar."

b.    "Just look at how upset your baby has become. Give him to me, and I'll feed him for you."

c.    "Your burping technique is good, but try burping him only at the end of the feeding."

d.    "He's confused, Mrs Paar. Put him on your shoulder to burp him."

50.    On your mother-baby unit, you are conducting mothers' classes on newborn characteristics. The mothers express concerns about the following common occurrences. How would you respond to each?

a.    "Can I hurt him by washing his hair over that soft spot? When will it close?"




b.    "All my family's eyes are brown, but her eyes are blue."




c.    "Why are there tiny white spots across the bridge of her nose and on her chin?"




d.    "Are my baby's eyes all right? There are bright red marks on the white part of his eyes."




e.    "He has white patches in his mouth. Is that milk? How can you determine the cause?"

f.   "My son's breasts are so swollen. Will the swelling go down?"

g.   "When I changed her diaper, there was blood on it."

h.   "Are her feet clubbed? They turn in."

i.   "Why does his head look funny? The bones of his head cross over each other and look so narrow on the sides."

j.   List other questions you have been asked by mothers and your responses to them.

# Circumcision

51.   Prior to discharge, Ryan is circumcised. What are your nursing responsibilities during and following the circumcision?

52.   Nursing interventions for Ryan following his circumcision include

    a.   administering an analgesic.

    b.   applying a topical anesthetic to the site.

    c.   keeping him in the nursery for 1 hour.

    d.   loosely wrapping the diaper around him.

53.    Michael, an uncircumcised newborn, is ready for discharge. What instructions should you give his mother about penile care?

# Discharge Teaching/Preparation for Care at Home

54.    You are to present a newborn discharge teaching program. List the essential components of this teaching program.

55.    The nurse is evaluating discharge teaching. Which statement by the parents demonstrates understanding of temperature assessment for an infant?

   a.   "Her temperature needs to be taken only when she shows signs of illness."

   b.   "We need to take her axillary temperature every day at home."

   c.   "We should only take her rectal temperature at home if she is sick enough to go to the doctor."

   d.   "She only needs to have her temperature taken when she feels warm to the touch."

56.    Nursing actions that help a new mother identify her own baby after birth include

   a.   calling the infant by name as soon as possible after birth.

   b.   feeding the infant the first few times so that the mother can see the procedure.

   c.   strongly encouraging the mother to breastfeed.

   d.   undressing the baby completely so that all body parts can be seen.

57.    Which of the following behaviors by a new father would indicate "engrossment"?

   a.   Being able to express disappointment about the sex of the child

   b.   Being afraid of hurting the infant while holding the infant

   c.   Noting the individual characteristics of the infant including molding

   d.   Stating that he feels more mature after seeing his infant for the first time

58.    Prior to discharge, what screening and immunizations procedures should be instituted?

59.    For the trip home from the birthing center, the newborn would be adequately protected if transported in

    a.    an appropriate car seat facing the rear of the car.

    b.    the mother's arms while she is seated in the rear of the car.

    c.    an infant carrier secured to the rear seat with a seat belt.

    d.    an approved car seat facing forward between two passengers in the rear seat.

60.    Briefly identify some culturally based newborn care practices that you have encountered or you have seen in your family.

61.    **Memory Check:** Define the following abbreviations.

    a.    AC

    b.    BAT

    c.    CC

    d.    HC

    e.    PKU

# Internet Resources

**http://www.lalecheleague.org**
Answers to frequently asked questions about breastfeeding can be found at the La Leche League International web site. The site includes many in-depth articles on lactation management.

TOPIC

# 14 Nursing Care of Newborns with Conditions Present at Birth

The majority of pregnancies end with the birth of healthy term infants. However some infants are at risk even before birth because of an altered intrauterine environment. In many instances the maternal or fetal factors that increase the baby's risk can be predicted during the antepartal period. Recognition of these factors and early nursing intervention can significantly improve the baby's outlook.

This topic first considers the factors that contribute to the development of an at-risk infant and the commonly used methods of assessing an infant's status. It then focuses on the problems these at-risk infants face.

This topic corresponds to Chapter 28 in the sixth edition of *Maternal-Newborn Nursing: A Family and Community-Based Approach*.

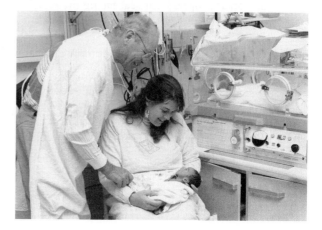

## Classification of At-Risk Infants

1. Identify six maternal factors that may contribute to the birth of an at-risk infant.

   a.

   b.

   c.

   d.

   e.

   f.

Using a neonatal classification and mortality chart, plot each newborn's gestational age and weight, and identify the appropriate classification for each of the following newborns (each newborn may belong to a classification group based on both gestational age and weight):

2.   Baby Joey is at 36–37 weeks' gestation, twin B, weighing 1500 g.

     Classification _____

3.   Baby Gwynn is at 42½ weeks' gestation by clinical determination and weighs 3150 g.

     Classification _____

4.   Baby Sara is 34 weeks and weighs 2060 g.

     Classification _____

5.   Baby Fernando is a 39-week newborn weighing 3950 g.

     Classification _____

6.   Baby Carla is 41 weeks and weighs 2500 g.

     Classification _____

7.   In assessing the newborn for at-risk status, the nurse should know that
   a.   any infant with a birth weight of less than 2500 grams is preterm.
   b.   the large-for-gestational-age infant has little risk of neonatal morbidity.
   c.   gestational age is the one criterion utilized to establish mortality risk.
   d.   infants who are preterm and small for gestational age have the highest mortality risk.

## Small-for-Gestational-Age (SGA) Infant

8.   List four maternal causes for an SGA infant.

   a.

   b.

   c.

   d.

9.    What physical findings would you expect when scoring the gestational age of an SGA infant?

10.    Describe the potential complications associated with an SGA infant.

# Infant of a Diabetic Mother (IDM)

11.    Richard is a 36 weeks' gestation newborn, weighing 9 lb, 1 oz. His admitting nursery information indicates that his mother is a class C diabetic. What physical characteristics would you expect him to have?

12.    Identify the cause for Richard's large size.

13.    What laboratory test should be carried out on Richard and when?

14.    Richard may show beginning signs of hypoglycemia _____ hours after birth.

15.    Hypoglycemia occurs when blood glucose levels fall below _____ mg/dL.

16.    What signs of developing hypoglycemia would you observe in Richard? (See Chapter 29.)

17.   Identify the nursing interventions you would carry out relative to the assessment and treatment of hypoglycemia.

18.   Richard is a newborn who experienced symptomatic hypoglycemia and required an intravenous infusion of dextrose. His condition has stabilized, and the physician has changed him to oral feedings. As Richard begins oral feedings, the nurse should anticipate that medical orders will include

    a.   discontinuing of IV after first formula feeding.

    b.   administering long-acting epinephrine.

    c.   giving a bolus infusion of 25-percent dextrose.

    d.   reinstituting frequent glucose monitoring during transition.

19.   Infants of diabetic mothers are at risk for which of the following problems?

    a.   Erythroblastosis fetalis

    b.   Hypercalcemia

    c.   Respiratory distress syndrome

    d.   Seizures

20.   Identify three other complications for which Richard is at risk.

## Postterm Infant

21.   List three obstetric indications of a postterm pregnancy.

    a.

    b.

    c.

22.    Describe the clinical picture of a postterm infant.

23.    Like the preterm infant, the newborn with postmaturity syndrome is at high risk for cold stress due to

  a.  extended posture.

  b.  absence of vernix.

  c.  parchment-like skin.

  d.  decreased subcutaneous fat.

24.    Describe the potential complications for a postterm infant.

# Preterm Infant

25.    List four major causes of prematurity.

  a.

  b.

  c.

  d.

26.    Which of the following characteristics is indicative of a preterm newborn of 34 weeks' gestation?

  a.  The scalp hair is silky and lies in silky strands

  b.  The skin, except for the face, is covered with lanugo

  c.  The sole creases cover the anterior two-thirds of the foot

  d.  The upper two-thirds of the pinna curves inward

27.    A preterm infant arrives in the nursery. What three initial assessments should you make?

a.

b.

c.

28.    When auscultating the chest of a preterm newborn the nurse hears rales and a continuous systolic murmur with clicks at the base of the heart. The nurse should suspect the presence of

a.    bronchopulmonary dysplasia.

b.    patent ductus arteriosus.

c.    pulmonary atelectasis.

d.    a ventricular septal defect.

29.    If an infant experiences an apneic episode, the first nursing activity should be to

a.    apply gentle tactile stimulation.

b.    call the physician.

c.    increase the rate of prescribed oxygen.

d.    suction the mouth and nose with a bulb syringe.

30.    The most common complication associated with preterm births is the development of

a.    bronchopulmonary dysplasia.

b.    periodic apnea.

c.    persistent fetal circulation.

d.    respiratory distress syndrome.

31.    Briefly describe the benefits of each: early breast-milk feedings (see Chapter 27) and premature formulas.

Mariah, a 34-week preterm infant, is initially maintained on intravenous fluids via umbilical catheter. When her respiratory status improves, she is placed on a half-strength premature formula via gavage feedings every 2 hours.

32.  List three methods of assessing proper placement of a gavage tube prior to feedings.

a.

b.

c.

33.  What nursing assessments would you make to determine the following?

a.  Mariah's tolerance of gavage feedings

b.  Mariah's readiness for nipple feeding

34.  When Mariah is two days old, her weight is average for gestational age (AGA). She is being carefully monitored prior to initiation of nipple feeding. Which of the following data groups would indicate that she is not ready for nipple feeding?

a.  Gaining weight; coordinated suck-swallow reflex

b.  Alert; axillary temperature of 97F

c.  Apical heart rate 120; skin temperature 36.5C

d.  Nasal flaring; sustained respiratory rate of 68

35.  Briefly describe developmentally supportive nursing measures.

36.    What would you do to facilitate attachment between parents and their at-risk infant?

37.    What observations would you make in assessing the readiness of Mariah's parents to take her home?

# Infant of Substance-Abusing Mother

38.    What common complications may be associated with cocaine-exposed infants?

39.    Claire, a 2-day-old, 3100-g newborn, is observed to be going through withdrawal. Her 18-year-old mother was addicted to heroin during the pregnancy. List six symptoms of withdrawal you may observe in Claire.

a.

b.

c.

d.

e.

f.

40.    The nursing management of a heroin-addicted newborn experiencing withdrawal includes

a.    administration of methadone and frequent assessment of vital signs.

b.    frequent assessment of vital signs and wrapping the infant snugly in a blanket.

c.    meticulous skin and perineal care and frequent tactile stimulation.

d.    minimal tactile stimulation and the provision of loose, nonrestrictive clothing.

41.    During the past week, Claire has been irritable and eating poorly. She has not gained weight since birth. The physician orders phenobarbital for her. How many milligrams will the nurse administer per dose?

a.    6 mg

b.    12 mg

c.    24 mg

d.    36 mg

42.    What are the special needs of the drug-exposed infant at home?

# Newborn at Risk for AIDS

43.    Nursing interventions for an infant at risk for AIDS include

a.    a quiet, dim environment.

b.    feeding with 24 cal/oz formula.

c.    frequent, gentle handling.

d.    tight swaddling.

44.    What instructions for care in the home should be given to parents of an infant at risk for AIDS?

---

## REFLECTIONS

Think about an at-risk newborn you have taken care of. What were the parents' responses? Describe what the experience was like for you.

_____

_____

_____

_____

_____

_____

_____

---

45.    John is a newborn at risk for AIDS. John's parents are very anxious when they see him with all the special equipment around him. Your best response to facilitate parent-infant interaction would be to

    a.    assure them that they are fortunate to have John in a special-care nursery.

    b.    explain the equipment in simple terms, have them wash their hands, and provide an opportunity for them to touch John.

    c.    explain the equipment simply and discuss the viability and continued existence of John.

    d.    have them wash their hands so they can touch John.

46.    **Memory Check:** Define the following abbreviations.

    a.    AIDS

    b.    FAE

    c.    FAS

d. IDM

e. ISAM

f. IUGR

g. LGA

h. SGA

# 15 Nursing Care of Newborns with Birth-Related Stressors

The majority of pregnancies end with the birth of healthy term infants. However, some infants develop serious problems during their early hours and days of life. In many instances the maternal or fetal factors that increase the baby's risk can be predicted during the antepartal period. In other cases the infant's risk status results from insults or complications that occur during labor and birth. In both instances early interventions can significantly improve the baby's outlook.

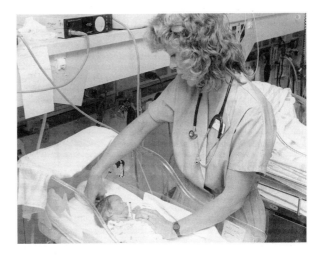

This topic focuses on many of the problems that may afflict high-risk infants, with emphasis on nursing assessment and interventions and, finally, on evaluation of effectiveness of care.

This topic also integrates content from prior newborn topics and corresponds to Chapter 29 in the sixth edition of *Maternal-Newborn Nursing: A Family and Community-Based Approach*.

## Resuscitation

Immediate newborn care for all at-risk newborns, in addition to providing warmth, is centered around determining the need for resuscitation.

1. Dawn Walker has a previous obstetric history of fetal death of undetermined cause at 8 months' gestation. After the physician obtains a fetal scalp blood pH of 7.22, baby boy Walker is born. Which action by the nurse is the appropriate *initial* newborn resuscitation step?

   a. Inserting a nasogastric tube

   b. Suctioning the oro- and nasopharynx

   c. Inflating the lungs with positive pressure

   d. Positioning the head in the "sniffing position"

2.  Baby Ken, a 43½-week postterm newborn, experienced early deceleration in labor. Yellow-green amniotic fluid was present at the time of membrane rupture.

    a.  Ken is at risk for what neonatal problem?

    b.  What resuscitative measures should be instituted as soon as his head and face appear on the perineum?

    c.  What additional resuscitative measures or actions do you anticipate will be carried out after Ken is born?

3.  **Critical Thinking Challenge:** The following situation has been included to challenge your critical thinking. Read the situation, then answer the question "yes" or "no," and give the rationale for your decision.

    Celeste, a 3200-g term baby, is born vaginally. The amniotic fluid is lightly meconium stained. She was suctioned on the perineum and cried vigorously within 30 seconds of birth.

    **Is Celeste a candidate for further resuscitation measures?**

    Yes _____                              No _____

    Explain your answer:

Brian, a term baby, was born vaginally 2 hours after his mother received 75 mg of Demerol IM. He has some flexion of extremities and acrocyanosis, a heart rate of 96, slow and irregular respiratory effort, and facial grimace. His Apgar at 1 min is 5. You are assisting the physician/neonatal nurse practitioner with the resuscitation.

4.   Why is deep, vigorous suctioning of the airways to be avoided?

5.   During bag-and-mask resuscitation you watch Brian's resuscitation bag to ensure it is inflating adequately, and you watch the pressure manometer to achieve the desired pressure of

(a) _____ cm $H_2O$ at a rate of (b) _____ times/min.

6.   Based on Brian's intrapartal history, what other resuscitative measures does he need?

7.   The first pharmacologic agent given in the chemical resuscitation phase of neonatal resuscitation is

a.   dopamine, to correct acidosis.

b.   epinephrine, to stimulate the heart.

c.   sodium bicarbonate, to correct acidosis.

d.   a volume expander, to maintain blood pressure.

On April 18 at 1:45 PM, a 35-week, 1580-g male infant named Julio was born to a 20-year-old primigravida.

8.   Julio is beginning to show signs of respiratory distress. Determine the priority for the following nursing interventions:

1.   Notify the physician.

2.   If cyanosis occurs, provide oxygen.

3.   Record time, symptoms, degree of symptoms, and whether oxygen relieved the symptoms of respiratory distress.

4.   Apply monitoring electrodes.

5.   Maintain a patent airway.

a.   2, 1, 5, 4, and 3

b.   5, 1, 2, 3, and 4

c.   4, 2, 5, 1, and 3

d.   5, 2, 1, 4, and 3

# Respiratory Distress Syndrome

Tricia, a 3½ lb (1587 g) newborn with a gestational age of 34 weeks, was born at 10:30 PM. Her Apgar score at 1 minute was 3, necessitating resuscitation via intubation and oxygen administration. On admission to the NICU, her vital signs are as follows: pulse 150, respirations 50, and rectal temperature of 96.2F (35.7C). She is placed in a radiant heat warmer, and an umbilical artery catheter is inserted for intravenous infusion.

9. You are to assess Tricia for signs of respiratory distress. List six signs indicative of developing respiratory distress.

   a.

   b.

   c.

   d.

   e.

   f.

10. Additional physical assessment data on Tricia's respiratory status reveal minimal nasal flaring, chest lag on inspiration with just visible intercostal (lower chest) and xiphoid retractions, and audible expiratory grunting. Using the Silverman-Andersen index (Figure 15–1), your respiratory distress score for Tricia would be _____.

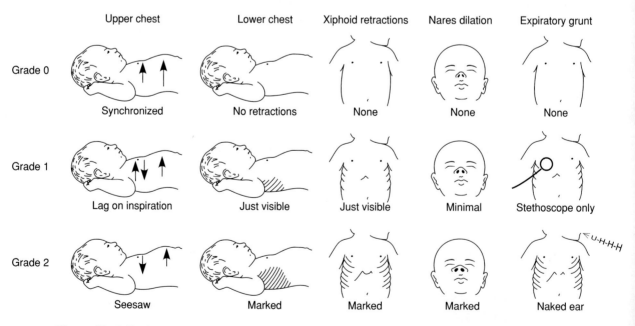

**Figure 15–1** Evaluation of respiratory status using the Silverman-Andersen index (from Ross Laboratories, Nursing Inservice Aid no. 2, Columbus, Ohio; and Silverman WA, Andersen DH: *Pediatrics* 1956:17:1. Copyright © 1956: American Academy of Pediatrics).

11.   What is the significance of Tricia's Silverman-Andersen score?

12.   What three factors may predispose Tricia to develop respiratory distress syndrome?

a.

b.

c.

13.   It is now 2 AM, and Tricia is showing signs of respiratory distress syndrome. She is placed in an oxygen hood with a warmed, humidified oxygen concentration of 70 percent. What is the rationale for administering warmed and humidified oxygen?

14.   Tricia's respirations are now 65 per minute; she has an apical pulse of 152–176 beats per minute; and her arterial blood gases show a pH of 7.3, $PO_2$ of 55 mm Hg, and $PCO_2$ of 69 mm Hg. What are your nursing responsibilities during oxygen administration and how can you evaluate the effectiveness of the oxygen therapy?

15. As Tricia's respiratory distress decreases, monitoring her respiratory status can be accomplished by noninvasive methods. Complete the following chart on noninvasive oxygen monitoring techniques.

| Technique | Action | Nursing Responsibilities |
|---|---|---|
| Transcutaneous oxygen monitor | | |
| Pulse oximeter | | |

16. Tricia's oxygen concentration is carefully regulated, based on her $PO_2$ and $PCO_2$ levels, because high blood levels of oxygen

    a. cause cardiac shunt closures, although the latter are not permanent.

    b. cause peripheral circulatory collapse.

    c. may cause retinal spasms, leading to the development of retinopathy of prematurity.

    d. may produce hyperbilirubinemia.

## Cold Stress

At-risk infants are susceptible to temperature instability and should be placed in a regulated neutral thermal environment. If the infant's thermal environment is not maintained, cold stress can occur.

17. What four metabolic changes and resultant problems may occur as a result of cold stress?

    a.

    b.

c.

d.

18. Describe the nursing interventions you would institute to prevent or minimize hypothermia/cold stress.

19. A small-for-gestational-age (SGA) newborn has experienced cold stress. Which of the following nursing actions should be included in the baby's care plan?
    a. Using radiant warmer, institute measures for rapid temperature elevation
    b. Initiate Dextrostix monitoring of blood glucose levels
    c. Monitor rectal temperature hourly
    d. Rapidly infuse 50-percent dextrose IV per standing protocol (or obtain order)

## Neonatal Jaundice

20. List three factors that influence the rate and amount of bilirubin conjugation.

    a.

    b.

    c.

21. State three situations that alter the newborn's ability to conjugate bilirubin.

    a.

    b.

    c.

22.    Identify the characteristics of pathologic jaundice as related to causes, time of onset, and bilirubin level in the term and preterm newborn.

23.    What factors might influence your assessment of the newborn's developing jaundice?

24.    An African-American mother asks how to assess for jaundice in her newborn. Which of the following is the most appropriate answer for the nurse to offer?

   a.    "A good place to look is the inside of the mouth. Use a good light to help you see."

   b.    "Pressing the sole of your baby's foot is helpful. If it blanches yellow, then the baby is considered jaundiced."

   c.    "The best way to assess your baby is to check the white part of the eyes. If jaundice is present, they will have a yellow color."

   d.    "Such an assessment is best done by the doctor. She knows how to identify jaundice."

25.    A newborn undergoing phototherapy experiences increased urine output and loose stools. The nurse should

   a.    institute enteric isolation.

   b.    immediately discontinue phototherapy.

   c.    decrease the phototherapy unit's level of irradiance.

   d.    observe for clinical manifestations of dehydration.

26.    While receiving phototherapy lights, babies should

   a.    be unclothed with the eyes shielded.

   b.    be unclothed with the eyes and genitals shielded.

   c.    not be removed from under the lights until treatment is completed.

   d.    not be disturbed by frequent parental visits.

27.    **Critical Thinking in Practice:** The following action sequence on page 217 is designed to help you think through a clinical problem pertaining to hemolytic disease of the newborn.

    You are taking care of Alice, a 24-hour-old, 7 lb, 2 oz newborn, and her mother on the mother-baby unit. During your initial assessments and care of Alice, you notice she looks yellow.

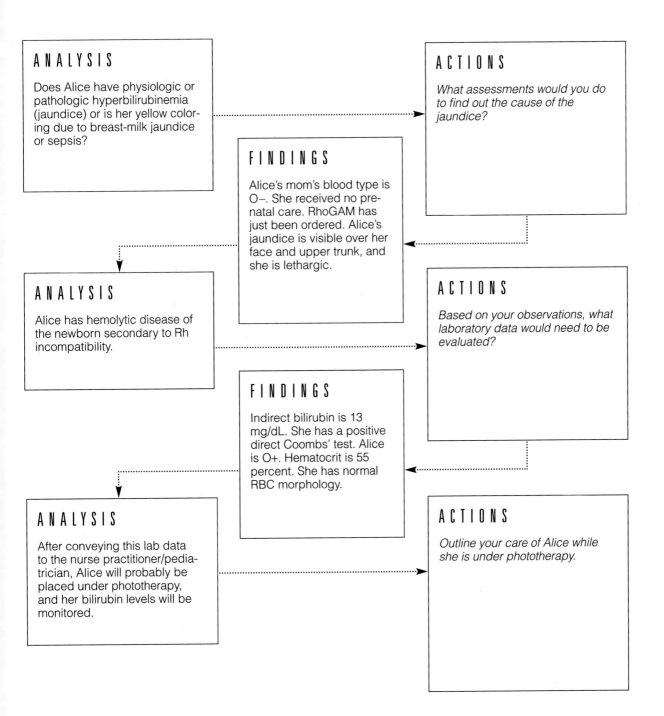

**ANALYSIS**

Does Alice have physiologic or pathologic hyperbilirubinemia (jaundice) or is her yellow coloring due to breast-milk jaundice or sepsis?

**ACTIONS**

*What assessments would you do to find out the cause of the jaundice?*

**FINDINGS**

Alice's mom's blood type is O–. She received no prenatal care. RhoGAM has just been ordered. Alice's jaundice is visible over her face and upper trunk, and she is lethargic.

**ANALYSIS**

Alice has hemolytic disease of the newborn secondary to Rh incompatibility.

**ACTIONS**

*Based on your observations, what laboratory data would need to be evaluated?*

**FINDINGS**

Indirect bilirubin is 13 mg/dL. She has a positive direct Coombs' test. Alice is O+. Hematocrit is 55 percent. She has normal RBC morphology.

**ANALYSIS**

After conveying this lab data to the nurse practitioner/pediatrician, Alice will probably be placed under phototherapy, and her bilirubin levels will be monitored.

**ACTIONS**

*Outline your care of Alice while she is under phototherapy.*

## Newborn with Polycythemia

28.   For a newborn with polycythemia, which of the following laboratory results would indicate that medical therapy is effective?

  a.   Central venous hematocrit of 70 percent

  b.   Central venous hematocrit of 55 percent

  c.   Venous hemoglobin of 25 g/dL

  d.   Serum calcium level of 8.0 mg/dL

## Neonatal Infections

29.   You are taking care of Haruko, who is 2 days old, and you note that he is increasingly lethargic and refuses to eat. He is diagnosed as having sepsis neonatorum. List four factors that increase the newborn's susceptibility to infections.

   a.

   b.

   c.

   d.

30.   Identify three bacterial organisms that may cause sepsis neonatorum.

   a.

   b.

   c.

31.   In newborns, an early sign of sepsis is
   a.   hypothermia.
   b.   hyperglycemia.
   c.   jitteriness.
   d.   tachycardia.

32.   Identify four diagnostic tests that might be done in a septic work-up.

   a.

   b.

   c.

   d.

33.    What are your nursing responsibilities while caring for a septic newborn? Include your rationale.

34.    The most common congenitally acquired viral infection is

    a.    cytomegalovirus.

    b.    herpes simplex virus.

    c.    syphilis.

35.    **Memory Check:** Define the following abbreviations.

    a.    BPD

    b.    MAS

    c.    RDS

    d.    TNZ

    e.    UAC

# TOPIC 16 Nursing Assessment and Care of the Postpartal Family

The postpartal period is a time of major physiologic and psychologic adaptations as the body completes its adjustment following childbirth. This topic begins with questions on theoretical data about common physiologic and psychologic changes. The remainder of the topic emphasizes clinical application of the nursing process in providing care for the postpartal family.

This topic corresponds to Chapters 30 and 31 in the sixth edition of *Maternal-Newborn Nursing: A Family and Community-Based Approach*.

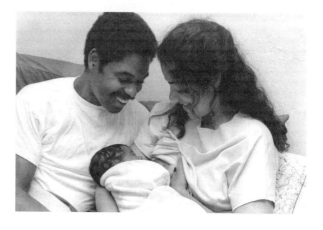

---

1.  Define *postpartum*.

## Attachment Immediately After Birth

2.  Lisa and George just had their first baby 10 minutes ago. What stage of labor and birth are they in?

3.  Lisa and George are exhibiting beginning attachment behaviors. What will you observe?

4.   How can you support the attachment process at this time?

# Physiologic Postpartal Changes

5.   The fundus should be

   a.   at the level of the symphysis pubis.

   b.   at the level of the umbilicus.

   c.   midway between the umbilicus and symphysis pubis.

   d.   two fingerbreadths below the umbilicus.

6.   The lochia should have a

   a.   characteristic foul odor and consist of blood mixed with a small amount of mucus.

   b.   characteristic foul odor and a dark brown color with occasional red bleeding.

   c.   fleshy odor and be clear-colored and moderate in amount.

   d.   fleshy odor with blood mixed in with a small amount of mucus.

7.   The perineum should be

   a.   edematous, painful to pressure, and displaying a clear discharge.

   b.   edematous, painful to pressure, and perhaps displaying hemorrhoids.

   c.   intensely painful in the episiotomy area and displaying clear drainage.

   d.   displaying clear drainage and perhaps hemorrhoids.

8.   The breasts should be

   a.   filling and secreting colostrum.

   b.   engorged and secreting colostrum.

   c.   soft and secreting milk.

   d.   engorged and not secreting any fluid.

9.   Uterine involution occurs as a result of

   a.   a decrease in the number of myometrial cells.

   b.   necrosis of the hypertrophic myometrial cells.

   c.   autolysis of protein material within the uterine wall.

   d.   necrotic degeneration of the placental site.

10.    Explain the physiologic mechanisms that cause each of the following:

   a.    Postpartal chill

   b.    Postpartal diaphoresis

   c.    Afterpains

11.    During the postpartal period, what psychologic adaptations does a new mother face?

12.    Describe "postpartum blues."

# Maternal Role Attainment

13.    Name and briefly describe the four stages of maternal role attainment.

   a.

   b.

c.

d.

## Assessment of the Postpartal Woman

14. Identify nine areas that should be examined during the initial postpartal *physical* assessment and then at least daily until the woman is discharged. (Do not include psychologic assessment or information needs.)

    a.

    b.

    c.

    d.

    e.

    f.

    g.

    h.

    i.

15. Describe three observations you should make in assessing the breasts of a woman postpartally. Include your rationale for each.

    a.

b.


c.


16.    The fundus is assessed following childbirth.

a.    Why is it necessary?


b.    Why is the client asked to empty her bladder before you assess her fundus?


c.    Describe the correct procedure for evaluating descent of the fundus.


d.    How is fundal height recorded (according to your agency's policy)?


17.    Soon Yee, a 21-year-old primipara, gave birth 4 hours ago. Immediately following birth her fundus was midway between the symphysis and the umbilicus. Where would you expect it to be now?


18.    What characteristics should you note in assessing Soon's lochia?


19.    How do you record your findings about her lochia (according to your agency's policy)?


20.    Soon reports that she got up to the bathroom a short time ago and noticed a sudden increase in her lochia. From your check you know that her fundus is firm. How would you explain this occurrence to her?

21.   In preparation for assessing Soon's perineum, you would have her assume the

   _____ position.

22.   What observations about the condition of the client's anal area should be made during the assessment of the perineum?

23.   What information regarding the client's urinary elimination should you elicit during your physical assessment?

24.   What information about your client's intestinal elimination should you elicit during your physical assessment?

25.   Discuss the teaching implications of your findings on intestinal elimination.

26.   Why is it important to include an evaluation of your client's lower extremities as part of your postpartal assessment?

27.   How is Homans' sign elicited?

28.   **Critical Thinking in Practice:** The following action sequence is designed to help you think through basic clinical problems.

Margo Jessup gave birth at 4:00 AM. At 8:30 AM you are completing her morning postpartum assessment. You find her fundus at one fingerbreadth above the umbilicus and displaced to the right side.

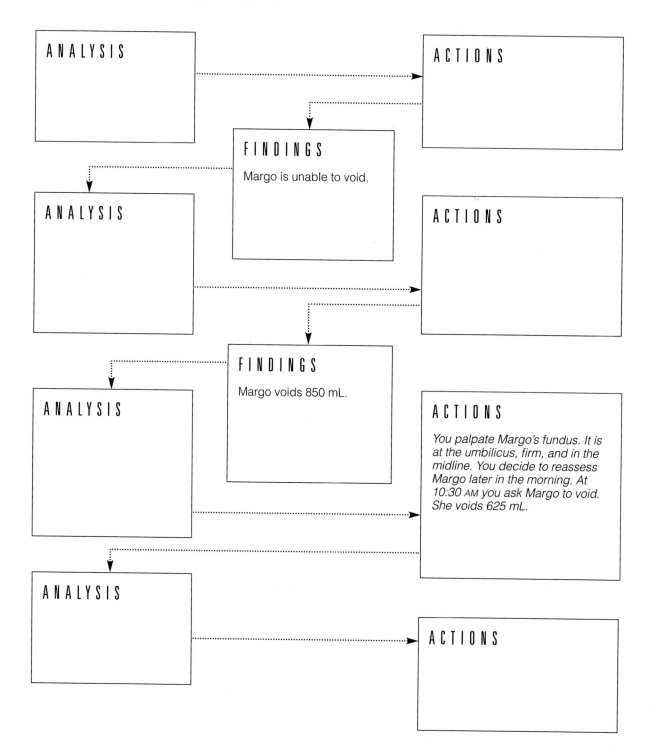

**FINDINGS**

Margo is unable to void.

**FINDINGS**

Margo voids 850 mL.

**ACTIONS**

You palpate Margo's fundus. It is at the umbilicus, firm, and in the midline. You decide to reassess Margo later in the morning. At 10:30 AM you ask Margo to void. She voids 625 mL.

# REFLECTIONS

Think about a woman you have cared for postpartally or someone you have visited soon after the birth of a child (perhaps this may apply to you). What were her emotions like? Did she share her feelings with you? Did she show any signs of the postpartum blues?

_____

_____

_____

_____

_____

_____

_____

_____

29.    What assessments are important in evaluating your client's nutritional status?

30.    Discuss factors you should consider in completing a psychologic assessment postpartally.

# Relief of Postpartal Discomforts

31.    For each of the discomforts listed below, identify two comfort measures.

    a.    Episiotomy

    b.    Hemorrhoids

    c.    Afterpains

# Suppression of Lactation

32.    Suppression of lactation in nonnursing mothers is generally accomplished by mechanical methods. Explain these methods.

33.    You are assisting Edna Lewis to the bathroom for the first time following childbirth.

    a.    What nursing assessments should you make before Edna gets up?

    b.    What teaching regarding perineal hygiene should you initiate at this time?

    c.    Edna decides to remain in the bathroom and take a shower after she voids. What precautions should you take to ensure her safety?

34.  During the postpartal period, you may be asked to administer a rubella vaccine. Describe the action/use, dose, side effects/untoward effects, and nursing considerations.

# Psychologic Responses

35.  Identify factors that influence a new mother's psychologic adjustment to childbirth and her newborn.

36.  How can a nurse provide emotional support during this time?

37.  You are caring for a woman who gave birth to a healthy infant 5 hours ago. When you enter her room, she is crying. She states, "I don't know what's wrong with me. I feel as let down as if it were the day after Christmas, and I can't seem to stop crying. What's going on? Do you know why I'm acting like this?" How would you respond?

38.  Freda and Earl Menzel express concern about the possible reaction of their 3-year-old son, Roy, to the birth of their daughter. Briefly describe some actions they might take to help Roy more easily adjust to the arrival of his sister.

39. In many postpartal units the focus of care and attention is the mother and her newborn. Describe how you would incorporate the father or support person into your focus of care.

40. In addition to her name, age, and social history, what information would you consider essential to have as part of your database in planning care for a woman postpartally?

41. Carla Jose, age 29, gravida, 3 para 2, gave birth to an 8 lb, 7 oz boy at 4:15 AM. Her labor lasted 18 hours, and the baby was born by low forceps. She received no medication during labor but did have a pudendal block for birth. She had a midline episiotomy and a third-degree extension. She also has two large hemorrhoids. The baby had an Apgar score of 7 at 1 minute and 9 at 5 minutes. He is apparently healthy, although he has a large bruise on each temple from the forceps and pronounced molding of his head. The labor nurse reported that Harry Jose, Carla's husband, was present at the birth and expressed great pleasure at the birth of his third son. Carla was openly disappointed that the newborn was not the girl she had so greatly desired.

It is now 8:00 AM. Carla has just finished breakfast, and you are assigned as her nurse today. Carla has voided twice since birth: 700 mL and 550 mL. Her fundus has remained firm and is at the umbilicus. Her lochia is rubra and moderate. Her vital signs are normal, and she is a breastfeeding mother. Her orders include a shower; a sitz bath tid, Dermaplast spray prn, up ad lib; Tylenol #3 q4h prn, a regular diet, fluids, a straight catheter × 1 prn for marked distention, and one capsule of Surfak bid. She is to be discharged at noon unless complications arise.

a. What do you consider the highest priorities in planning Carla's physical care?

b. What behaviors might Carla exhibit that would suggest possible failure to attach?

## Postpartal Care of the Woman Following Cesarean Birth

42.    How does postpartum assessment and care differ for the woman who gives birth by cesarean?

43.    Patient-controlled analgesia (PCA) is used for pain control.

   a.    Describe how it is used.

   b.    How is the client on PCA protected from overdose?

## Care of the Adolescent Mother

44.    Describe some of the special nursing needs of the adolescent mother postpartally.

45.    How can the postpartum nurse provide support and assistance to a woman who is relinquishing her infant?

# Discharge Teaching

46.    Vicky and Larry Darnell are preparing to take their first child, Lori, home at 2:00 PM. Vicky is planning to bottle-feed Lori. Vicky had an uncomplicated labor and birth but has a small midline episiotomy that has caused some discomfort. You are assigned to Vicky today and are responsible for discharge teaching. Describe what information you will include in your discharge teaching for the following areas:

   a.    Care of the episiotomy

   b.    Rest

   c.    Activity and exercises

   d.    Resumption of sexual activity and birth control methods

   e.    Symptoms in the mother that should be reported

   f.    Support systems

g.  Baby care

h.  Symptoms in the baby that should be reported

i.  Infant safety (crib, car seat)

j.  Follow-up medical care for both mother and infant

k.  Community resources

47.  LaTisha Carson gave birth to her first child in the birthing room 6 hours ago. Now she is preparing for discharge. Describe how you will explain the reasons for and importance of returning to the hospital for a test for phenylketonuria and other metabolic disorders.

# TOPIC

# 17 Home Care of the Postpartal Family

Home care is an important component of childbearing nursing practice. The mother and newborn have been stabilized, and the parents have had opportunities to establish their beginning family in the birth center or hospital. However, the mother and newborn will continue to have significant physiological adjustments over the first few weeks, and family learning needs tend to increase. The whole family will continue to make changes and adjustments as they incorporate their first child or assist siblings with welcoming a sister or brother. The home provides a rich opportunity for assessment and teaching. The parents are in their own setting, and the nurse is able to tailor teaching and nursing care specifically for each family.

This topic emphasizes continued assessment, anticipated findings and their significance, and appropriate nursing interventions. Questions related to evaluation are also included to provide guidelines for determining the effectiveness of care.

This topic corresponds to Chapter 32 in *Maternal-Newborn Nursing: A Family and Community-Based Approach*, sixth edition.

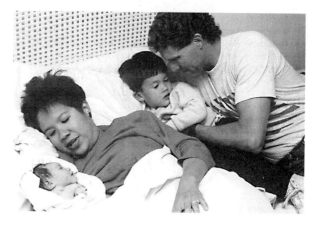

## Home Visits

1. The three areas of focus for a home visit to a postpartal family include

   a.

   b.

   c.

2. How is a postpartal home visit different from community health visits?

3.    Identify five actions a nurse should take to ensure personal safety during a home visit.

a.

b.

c.

d.

e.

4.    What should the nurse do if he or she begins to feel unsafe during a home visit?

# Home Care of the Newborn

5.    Which of the following holding methods is recommended when shampooing the infant?
a.    Cradle hold
b.    Football hold
c.    Upright position

6.    Why should the infant's resting position be changed periodically, especially during the early months of life?

7.    Identify at least two reasons for positioning a newborn infant on her or his side in the first week of life.

a.

b.

8. You are on a home visit to Elena Espinoza and her newborn daughter, Rose. Elena asks when she can switch from sponge baths to tub baths. How would you respond?

9. What information should you give Elena about assessment and care of Rose's umbilical cord?

10. The newborn's temperature should be taken by the _____ route.

For each of the following statements about newborn care, indicate **T** if the statement is true and **F** if it is false.

11. _____ Newborns should be given a daily bath.

12. _____ The eyes are washed from the inner to the outer canthus.

13. _____ The ear canal should be cleaned regularly with a cotton swab.

14. _____ Talcum powder is applied generously to help keep the infant's skin dry.

15. _____ The genital area should be cleansed daily with soap and water and with water after each wet or dirty diaper.

16. _____ The foreskin of uncircumcised infants should be gently retracted each day.

17. _____ If necessary, the newborn's nails may be trimmed straight across.

18.   Complete the following chart comparing the stools of breastfed and formula-fed infants.

| Characteristics of Stools | Breastfed | Formula-Fed |
| --- | --- | --- |
| Frequency | | |
| Color | | |
| Consistency | | |
| Odor | | |

# Home Care of the Postpartal Woman and Family

19.   List four physical and developmental tasks the new mother must accomplish during the post-partal period.

   a.

   b.

   c.

   d.

20.   Summarize areas of assessment the nurse should complete on the new mother during a postpartal home visit.

   a.   Physical assessment

   b.   Psychosocial assessment

For each of the following physical findings in the postpartal woman, indicate with a "**1**" those that are normally found at the first postpartal home visit and with a "**6**" those that are normally found by six weeks postpartum.

21. _____ Weight loss of 30 lb

22. _____ Abdominal musculature somewhat lax

23. _____ Striae pink and readily apparent

24. _____ Nonnursing mother: breasts firm to the touch

25. _____ Normal bowel elimination pattern

26. _____ Lochia serosa, scant

27. _____ Fundus not palpable above symphysis

28. During a home visit, you assess a new mother for signs of bonding with her infant. List at least five signs that might indicate a failure to bond.

    a.

    b.

    c.

    d.

    e.

# Support for the Breastfeeding Mother

29. The mother states she is having difficulty with breastfeeding. How might you help her?

# Internet Resources

**http://www.brightfutures.org**
Bright Futures' web site has extensive information on infancy (0–12 months) home care. Explanations of expected prenatal, newborn, and second- to ninth-month development are described in detail.

# TOPIC 18

# The Postpartal Family at Risk

The postpartal period is regarded by some as rather anticlimactic. After even the most uneventful birth, nursing assessments of mother and baby are essential, especially in light of the recent trend of early discharge. The emotional support and teaching a postpartal nurse provides cannot be overemphasized, nor can the nurse's responsibility to carefully monitor the mother's physical status. Complications do sometimes develop in the birthing center or at home during the postpartal period, but their severity may often be ameliorated by early detection and interaction.

This topic corresponds to Chapter 33 in the sixth edition of *Maternal-Newborn Nursing: A Family and Community-Based Approach*.

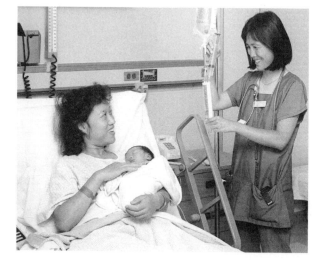

## Postpartum Hemorrhage

1. Postpartum hemorrhage may be classified as early or late. Describe the time of onset and primary cause(s) of each.

   a. Early

   b. Late

Joan Taranta, a 33-year-old gravida 3, para 3, is recovering following the birth of twin boys. Her labor lasted 2½ hours.

2. Identify two factors that predispose Joan to early postpartum hemorrhage.

   a.

   b.

3.    During your assessment of Joan, what three findings would indicate possible postpartum hemorrhage?

    a.

    b.

    c.

4.    Your nursing assessment indicates that Joan is having an early postpartum hemorrhage. Formulate an appropriate nursing diagnosis.

5.    What do you consider the two highest priorities in planning your care of Joan?

6.    The nurse finds Joan's uterus to be boggy, high, and deviated to the right. The most appropriate nursing action is to

    a.    have Joan void and then reevaluate the fundus.

    b.    massage the uterus and reevaluate it in 30 minutes.

    c.    notify the physician.

    d.    place Joan on a pad count.

7.    What additional nursing interventions should be initiated for Joan as she demonstrates signs of postpartum hemorrhage?

8.  A client who has an estimated blood loss of 1300 mL 8 hours postbirth is said to have

    a.  mild, early postpartum hemorrhage.

    b.  severe, early postpartum hemorrhage.

    c.  mild, late postpartum hemorrhage.

    d.  severe, late postpartum hemorrhage.

9.  **Critical Thinking in Practice:** The following action sequence is designed to help you think through basic clinical problems.

    You are taking care of Mrs Carrie Spencer, age 24, gravida 1, para 1, on the mother-baby unit. She is 8 hours postbirth of an 8 lb, 2 oz baby girl. As you are carrying out her postpartal assessments, she complains of tenderness and pain in her perineal area. She says, "My stitches hurt; it feels as if they are tearing apart."

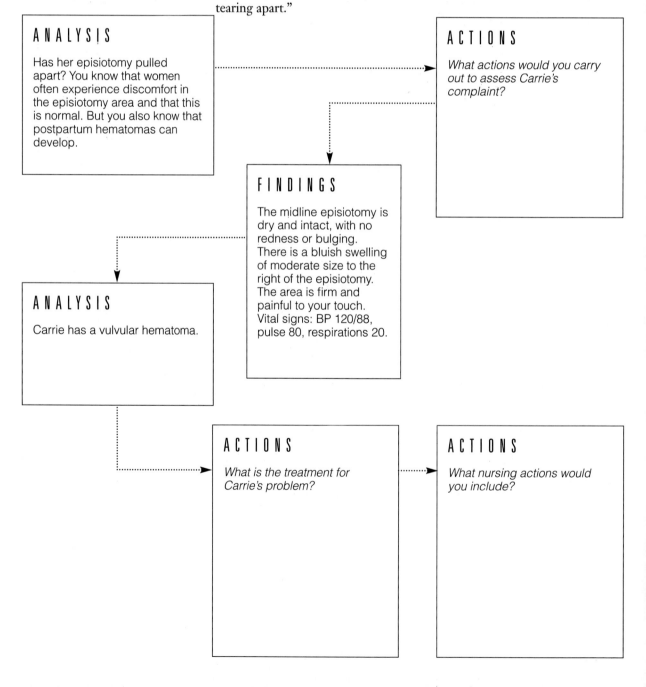

ANALYSIS

Has her episiotomy pulled apart? You know that women often experience discomfort in the episiotomy area and that this is normal. But you also know that postpartum hematomas can develop.

ACTIONS

*What actions would you carry out to assess Carrie's complaint?*

FINDINGS

The midline episiotomy is dry and intact, with no redness or bulging. There is a bluish swelling of moderate size to the right of the episiotomy. The area is firm and painful to your touch. Vital signs: BP 120/88, pulse 80, respirations 20.

ANALYSIS

Carrie has a vulvular hematoma.

ACTIONS

*What is the treatment for Carrie's problem?*

ACTIONS

*What nursing actions would you include?*

## Subinvolution

Mrs Gloria Brown, a breastfeeding mother, gave birth to a 8 lb, 11½ oz baby boy, Vincent, vaginally after Pitocin augmentation. She has been home for 2 weeks and calls the office. She tells the ob/gyn nurse practitioner that she is concerned because her flow has increased and is red but not foul smelling.

10.   Identify nursing assessments that might lead you to suspect subinvolution.

11.   Identify three nursing interventions to meet Gloria's needs.

## Postpartal Reproductive Tract Infections

12.   Identify the physiologic reasons why a woman during labor and birth has an increased suscep-
      tibility to infection.

      a.

      b.

      c.

      d.

13.   The clinical manifestations of a localized infection of the episiotomy would include

      a.   approximation of the skin edges of the episiotomy.

      b.   client complaint of severe discomfort in the perineum and an oral temperature of 99.8F
           (37.7C).

      c.   reddened, bruised tissue.

      d.   reddened, edematous tissue with yellowish discharge.

Rich and Kim Ayyad have delivered their third baby by cesarean birth.

14.   The nurse's assessment of Kim reveals an elevation in her temperature, chills, nausea, and
      increased pain. The nurse notifies the primary physician and receives the following orders:
      500 mg of ampicillin by IV q6h, culture and sensitivity of lochia, ultrasound of the pelvis,
      and a chest x-ray. Which order should the nurse carry out first?

      a.   Ultrasound

      b.   IV antibiotic

      c.   Culture of lochia

      d.   Chest x-ray

15.    Kim's incision has become infected, and she has been placed in isolation. Since the baby can no longer room-in, how can the nurse promote bonding between Kim and her infant?

a.    Provide a picture of the baby for Kim.

b.    Have Rich visit the baby more often.

c.    Assure Kim she will be in isolation only a short time.

d.    Encourage Kim to use the time away from the baby to rest so she will recover faster.

16.    Complete the following chart on puerperal infection:

| Component | Localized Infection (Episiotomy and/or Laceration) | Endometritis (Metritis) | Pelvic Cellulitis (Parametritis) |
|---|---|---|---|
| Tissues involved | | | |
| Clinical manifestations | | | |
| Interventions | | | |
| Complications | | | |

17.    Identify evaluative outcome criteria findings that indicate your interventions/treatments of the puerperal infection have been effective.

18.    What home care instructions would you give a mother about puerperal infections?

19.   **Critical Thinking Challenge:** The following situation has been included to challenge your critical thinking. Read the situation, answer the question "yes" or "no," and give your rationale.

Jeanne McGuire, age 34, gravida 3, para 3, gave birth to twin boys vaginally with regional anesthesia 12 hours ago and you are now responsible for her care. She complains of cramping when the uterus attempts to contract. Your assessment reveals a uterus one fingerbreadth above the umbilicus and displaced to the right, and increased vaginal bleeding.

**Is Jeanne a candidate for bladder distention?**

Yes _____                    No _____

Explain your answer:

## Puerperal Cystitis

20.   List three factors that predispose the postpartal woman to the development of cystitis.

a.

b.

c.

21.   Identify appropriate interventions in the treatment of the postpartal woman with cystitis.

# Mastitis

One week after her discharge, Alice Enriquez, a 23-year-old gravida 1, para 1, breastfeeding mother, develops mastitis.

22.    List two factors that contribute to the development of mastitis.

   a.

   b.

23.    Identify four clinical manifestations of mastitis that Alice may exhibit.

   a.

   b.

   c.

   d.

Two nursing diagnoses that may apply to Alice are *Acute Pain* related to inflammation and swelling of breast tissue and *Knowledge Deficit* related to lack of information about appropriate breastfeeding techniques.

24.    Based on these possible nursing diagnoses, describe the interventions that Alice or you may institute.

25.    In evaluating the nursing diagnosis *Knowledge Deficit* related to lack of information about appropriate breastfeeding techniques, identify the evaluative outcome criteria that would indicate that Alice's knowledge about breastfeeding during mastitis has changed.

# Thromboembolic Diseases

26.   Discuss the physiologic changes of pregnancy that increase a woman's susceptibility to blood clot formation during the postpartal period.

Match the following descriptive statements with the correct thromboembolic disease.

27. _____   Clotting process involving the saphenous vein system

28. _____   More frequently seen in women with history of thrombosis

29. _____   Usually appears about the third or fourth postpartal day

30. _____   Sudden onset of sweating, pallor, dyspnea, and chest pain

31. _____   Prompt intervention with heparin, oxygen, and lidocaine as needed

32. _____   Edema of ankle and leg; low-grade fever and positive Homans' sign

33. _____   Treatment primarily involves intravenous heparin and bed rest

34. _____   Management principally involves leg elevation, moist packs, bed rest, and elastic stockings

a.   Superficial thrombophlebitis

b.   Deep vein thrombosis (DVT)

c.   Pulmonary embolism

35.   Identify three interventions useful in preventing the development of thrombophlebitis during the postpartal period.

a.

b.

c.

36.    Describe the appropriate interventions for a mother with deep vein thrombosis.

Marie LaCoste has recently given birth and states that she has a history of thrombophlebitis.

37.    Which of the following nursing measures will be most important for Marie in light of her history?

   a.    Assess vital signs frequently

   b.    Encourage early ambulation

   c.    Encourage Marie to rest in bed with the knee gatch up

   d.    Maintain bed rest

38.    Marie has developed thrombophlebitis and is receiving heparin intravenously. It will be important to watch her for signs of overdose, which include

   a.    dysuria.

   b.    epistaxis, hematuria, and dysuria.

   c.    hematuria, ecchymosis, and epistaxis.

   d.    hematuria, ecchymosis, and vertigo.

39.    The antagonist of heparin is ＿＿＿＿＿＿＿＿＿＿＿.

40.    A positive Homans' sign is indicated by a complaint of pain in

   a.    the foot when the client stands.

   b.    the leg when the foot is dorsiflexed while the knee is held flat.

   c.    the leg when the knee is flexed and the foot is extended.

   d.    the leg when the knee is held flat and the foot is rotated.

41.    What education for self-care at home should be given to a woman receiving warfarin (Coumadin)?

## Postpartal Mood Disorders

It is the third postpartal day for Bonnie Sumpter, an 18-year-old primipara. She is single and is keeping her baby. The nurse makes a home visit and expresses concern that Bonnie may not be bonding appropriately with her infant.

42.   Identify four feelings or behaviors that might indicate "postpartum blues."

   a.

   b.

   c.

   d.

## Internet Resources

**http://parsons.ab.umd.edu/~datkins/nurs669**
The Parsons web site was produced for the School of Nursing at the University of Maryland at Baltimore. A section on the postpartum period covers complications such as thrombophlebitis, peritonitis, mastitis, and depression.

# Epilogue

By now you are probably almost finished with your maternity rotation. We hope this workbook has helped you focus your study so that you are more comfortable in relating your knowledge of theory to your clinical practice. We believe that in this way you will be better nurses, and that the childbearing families for whom you are responsible will receive better care.

# 1 Answer Key

1. Answers include the following: partner and family in the labor room with the laboring woman; newborns in the room with their mothers during the postpartum period; siblings allowed to visit the maternity unit; fathers able to be actively involved in the labor and birth process; availability of family choices about the labor and birth (place of birth, primary care giver, birth-related experiences); shortened length of stay for the new mother and her infant.

2. The Act provides a postpartum stay of up to 48 hours following vaginal birth and up to 96 hours following cesarean birth at the discretion of the new mother and her health care provider.

3. (a) The professional nurse has graduated from a basic, accredited program in nursing, has successfully passed the NCLEX nursing examination and is licensed as a registered nurse; (b) the CNS has a master's degree and specialized knowledge and competence in a specific clinical area; (c) the NP has received specialized education in a master's degree program or certificate program and can function in an advanced practice role; (d) the CNM is educated as both a nurse and a midwife and is certified by the American College of Nurse-Midwives.

4. b

5. Health promotion, illness prevention, and individual responsibility

6. community-based

7. (a) Provides opportunity for additional support and teaching following discharge from an acute care setting; (b) enables people to remain at home with conditions that formerly would have required hospitalization.

8. See text, pp. 9–10

9. See text, pp. 14–15

10. (a) Number of live births per 1000 people; (b) number of deaths of infants under 1 year of age per 1000 live births in a given population; (c) number of deaths of infants less than 28 days of age per 1000 live births; (d) number of deaths from any cause during the pregnancy cycle (including the 42-day postpartal period) per 100,000 live births.

11. Answers include the following: increased use of hospitals and specialized health care personnel by maternity clients; improved high-risk care for mothers and infants; prevention and control of infection with antibiotics and improved techniques; availability of blood and blood products for transfusions; lowered rates of anesthesia-related deaths.

12. d

13. See text, pp. 22–26

# Answer Key

1. b
2. a
3. c
4. e
5. f
6. d
7. See text, p. 43
8. b
9. a
10. b
11. a
12. a and b
13. (a) 4, (b) 6
14. IUDs are recommended only for women who have given birth to a child and who are in a mutually monogamous sexual relationship. Until Marcella is sure that the relationship will be long-term and that the man is not sexually active with multiple partners, she is safer choosing another method of contraception; regardless of the method, she should insist that her partner use a condom.
15. (a) vasectomy, (b) tubal ligation
16. d
17. Monthly
18. Not recommended at this age for low-risk women
19. Annually
20. Annually
21. Annually
22. (a) inspection of the vulva; (b) inspection of the the vagina and cervix using a speculum; (c) bimanual examination (palpation) of the cervix, uterus, and ovaries.
23. All women have breasts that vary slightly in size and contour, but inspection helps a woman know her own breasts so that she can recognize changes. Changes in the way her breasts move or point as she moves them through a variety of positions can be significant. Moving the arms varies the pull on the skin and muscle of the chest so that masses or changes that are not visible in one position may become evident in another position.
24. See text, p. 54
25. d
26. Information Mrs Sanchez would benefit from includes the following self-care measures: the use of a fan and/or increased intake of cold liquids for the hot flashes, continued calcium supplementation, and use of water-soluble jelly during intercourse to counteract vaginal atrophy (increased frequency of intercourse also will maintain some elasticity in the vagina if this is an area of concern for her). It may also be of value to Mrs Sanchez to discuss other physical and emotional responses that may occur in menopause.
27. If you answered "yes," you are correct. Congratulations. Ms Swenson has several factors that place her at increased risk for osteoporosis, including early onset of menopause, fair complexion, slender build, and history of smoking.
28. (a) progestin, (b) endometrial cancer
29. d
30. d
31. a
32. e
33. You would probably mention simple practices such as limiting sodium intake and wearing a supportive bra. For more severe discomfort, the woman may ask her care giver for a prescription for a mild diuretic and might also use an over-the-counter analgesic. Even though controversy exists about the effectiveness of limiting methylxanthines (found in caffeine products), it can't hurt, and many women feel it is helpful. If you give the woman this information, she can then choose whether she wishes to try it. Other approaches include the use of thiamine and vitamin E. Use this time to stress the importance of monthly breast self-examination,

annual examinations by her health care provider, and regular mammograms as recommended by her health care provider.

34. (a) pelvic pain, (b) dyspareunia, (c) abnormal uterine bleeding

35. We hope you would discuss her medication in detail with her. It is important to review the purpose of the medication and possible side effects. You should also be certain that she clearly understands the dosage and administration schedule. In many instances women take danazol for a specified period of time (from three to eight months or longer), depending on the severity of the disease and the presence of palpable lesions. If she is scheduled to return for reevaluation at specified times, it is important that she understand the purpose and significance of these evaluations. Answer any questions she might have and give her an opportunity to voice any concerns about the therapy. If this medication is prescribed frequently in your office, you may want to develop a handout on it for clients to refer to when they are at home.

36. b

37. Your recommendations should include the following: Women with a history of TSS should *never* use tampons; others should avoid prolonged use of tampons, change tampons every 3–6 hours, avoid superabsorbent tampons, avoid overnight use of tampons, alternate tampons with sanitary napkins or minipads, and avoid tampon use for 6–8 weeks after childbirth. In addition, women should avoid leaving diaphragms or cervical caps in place for extended periods of time and never use them postpartally or when menstruating. They should also be aware of the signs of TSS.

38. c

39. a

40. b

41. a

42. d

43. c

44. a

45. b

46. *Actions:* In making your assessment it would be helpful to ask Nita whether she has noticed any change in her vaginal discharge. If she has, ask her to describe it. Because of the relationship between antibiotic therapy and monilial infection, you would ask whether she had been on antibiotics for any reason. It is always useful to ask clients whether they attribute the symptoms to anything. You may gain useful information about the condition or information about the client's perceptions.
*Analysis:* Based on the information obtained, you suspect that Nita has vulvovaginal candidiasis (VVC).
*Actions:* You tell Nita that, based on her symptoms, you suspect that she may have a yeast infection called vulvovaginal candidiasis. You point out that sometimes when women take antibiotics to destroy a bacterial infection, the antibiotics also destroy the normal, good bacteria found in a woman's vagina. When this happens, other organisms, especially yeast, may grow unchecked. You tell Nita that you will report your findings to the nurse practitioner (NP). You point out that the NP will probably do a vaginal examination and a test to confirm the infection type.
*Actions:* You would briefly describe Nita's symptoms and the appearance of her vaginal discharge and report the recent antibiotic therapy. You would say that you suspect that Nita might have VVC and ask the NP if she/he planned to do a vaginal examination and wet prep.
*Analysis:* Congratulations! Your analysis of the data was accurate. Hyphae and spores indicate VVC. Give yourself a pat on the back, too, for working in a collegial fashion with the NP.

47. Warn Marcy that she and her partner should avoid drinking alcohol while taking metronidazole because the combination has an effect similar to that of alcohol and Antabuse, including abdominal pain, flushing, and tremors.

48. infertility

49. See text, pp. 75–77

50. d

51. See text, p. 83

52 Answers may include the following: longer life expectation of women; the fact that older women tend to have less educational preparation than

older men; many women are economically dependent on men and may have intermittent or nonexistent employment histories; women typically earn less than men; women often work in jobs without pension benefits or only limited benefits; women generally have more family care-giving responsibilities than older men; women, more often than men, feel the impact of public policies and programs that place undue financial pressures on them.

53. See text, pp. 85–86
54. Occupational Safety and Health Administration
55. OSHA is responsible for creating and enforcing workplace health and safety regulations.
56. National Institute for Occupational Safety and Health
57. NIOSH is primarily a research agency, but it also disseminates information on preventing workplace injury and illness, provides training to occupational safety and health professionals, and investigates potentially hazardous working situations when requested by employers or employees.
58. See text, pp. 92–94

59. Methods used to exert power and control by one individual over another in an adult intimate relationship. Because 95 percent of the victims are women, this is also termed female partner abuse.
60. One; three
61. (a) Have you ever been emotionally or physically abused by your partner or someone close to you? (b) Within the last year, have you been hit, slapped, kicked, or otherwise physically hurt by someone?
62. Since you've been pregnant, have you been hit, slapped, kicked, or otherwise physically hurt by someone?
63. See text, p. 108
64. c
65. a
66. b
67. d
68. See text, p. 113
69. (a) basal body temperature, (b) breast self-examination, (c) Centers for Disease Control and Prevention, (d) dilatation & curettage, (e) fibrocystic breast disease, (f) pelvic inflammatory disease, (g) sexually transmitted disease, (h) urinary tract infection

# Answer Key

1. a
2. c
3. b
4. e
5. f
6. d
7. See text, p. 126, Figure 6–4
8. The vagina serves as a passageway for sperm, fetal delivery, and the products of menstruation. It protects against trauma from sexual intercourse and infection.
9. Factors that can destroy the self-cleansing ability of the vagina include antibiotic therapy, douching, and use of perineal sprays or deodorants.
10. (a) isthmus of fallopian tube, (b) uterine cavity, (c) uterine body, (d) endometrium, (e) myometrium, (f) internal os, (g) isthmus, (h) cervix, (i) vagina
11. b
12. The endometrium produces a thin, watery, alkaline secretion that helps sperm travel to the fallopian tubes; it nourishes the developing embryo prior to implantation.
13. (a) Lubricates vaginal canal, (b) acts as a bacteriostatic action, (c) provides an alkaline environment to protect sperm from the acidic vagina
14. b
15. See text, pp. 130–131
16. The fallopian tubes provide transport for the ovum from the ovary to the uterus (which takes three to four days); a site for fertilization; and a warm, moist, nourishing environment for the ovum and zygote.
17. See text, pp. 130–131
18. See text, p. 132
19. The ovaries secrete estrogen and progesterone and are responsible for ovulation.
20. See text, p. 130, 132–133, Figure 6–11
21. See text, p. 134, Figure 6–12
22. levator ani

23. (a) Portion above pelvic brim or linea terminalis; supports the pregnant uterus; directs the presenting fetal part into the true pelvis below. (b) Lies below the linea terminalis; its shape and size determine the adequacy of the birth passage. (c) Upper border of the true pelvis; usually rounded; determines whether engagement can occur. (d) Lower border of the true pelvis; if too narrow the baby's head may be pushed backward, making extension difficult and causing shoulder dystocia for large babies.
24. (a) false pelvis, (b) true pelvis, (c) pelvic inlet, (d) pelvic outlet
25. See text, p. 138, Figure 6–16
26. The tubercles of Montgomery secrete a fatty substance that helps lubricate and protect the breasts.
27. a
28. (a) ovarian, (b) menstrual
29. See text, pp.139–141
30. c
31. a
32. *Follicular phase:* under the influence of FSH, the graafian follicle matures; LH assists the oocyte in rupturing out of the ovary around day 14. *Luteal phase:* after rupture, the corpus luteum (CL) forms; if fertilization does not occur, the CL degenerates and progesterone and estrogen decrease, which results in menses.
33. See text, pp. 142–144
34. See text, p. 139, Figure 6–18
35. See text, pp. 142, 144
36. a
37. (a) penis, (b) epididymides, (c) vas deferens, (d) testes, (e) testis, (f) Leydig's cells, (g) seminiferous tubules, (h) Sertoli's, (i) seminal vesicles, (j) ejaculatory duct, (k) prostate, (l) seminal fluid, (m) bulbourethral (Cowper's)
38. (a) female reproductive cycle, (b) follicle-stimulating hormone, (c) gonadotropin-releasing hormone, (d) luteinizing hormone

# 4 Answer Key

1. *Mitosis:* Process to reproduce all body cells so that each cell is an exact replica of the original cell. *Meiosis:* A two-stage division process that ends with each cell having only half the number (23) of chromosomes of other body cells; process of replication for ovum and sperm only.

2. (a) 24, (b) 72

3. (a) 23, (b) 46

4. (a) XY, (b) male

5. b

6. See text, pp. 154–155

7. (a) Capacitation removes the sperm's plasma membrane and induces an attraction to the ovum. (b) Acrosomal reaction releases enzymes that break down the hyaluronic acid in the corona radiata, thereby allowing a single sperm to penetrate and fertilize the ovum.

8. a

9. c

10. d

11. e

12. b

13. (a) 7, (b) 9; Trophoblasts attach themselves to the endometrium for nourishment, the blastocyst burrows beneath the uterine lining which then thickens below the blastocyst, and the trophoblastic cells grow into the lining and form villi.

14. b

15. c

16. (a) chorion, (b) amnion

17. 350 mL at 20 weeks; after 20 weeks, amniotic fluid ranges from 700–1000 mL; the fluid is slightly alkaline and contains albumin, uric acid, creatinine, lecithin, sphingomyelin, bilirubin, vernix, leukocytes, epithelial cells, enzymes, and lanugo.

18. (a) decidua vera, (b) decidua basalis, (c) chorion, (d) amnion, (e) decidua capsularis

19. See text, p. 160

20. For the process through which the placenta develops, see text, p. 00. The maternal side appears red and fleshlike and is made up of the decidua basalis and its circulation. The fetal side appears shiny and gray and consists of the chorionic villi and their circulation; the placenta at term weighs 400–600 g, and its diameter is 15–20 cm (5.9–7.9 in).

21. Answers may include metabolic, transport, endocrine, immunologic.

22. See text, p. 165

23. The significant observations that you would want to make about the placenta would include determining the presence of all cotyledons, the presence of large infarcts or clots in the placenta, and the site of the umbilical insertion on the placenta. These observations will give you clues to potential problems for the newborn. The absence of cotyledons would indicate a need to have the clinician check the mother for retained placental fragments that could cause postpartum hemorrhage later.

24. (a) The embryonic stage starts on day 15 and continues until approximately the eighth week or until the embryo reaches a crown-rump (c-r) length of 3 cm or 1.2 inches. (b) By the end of the eighth week, every organ system and all external structures are present.

25. (a) 1, (b) 2, (c) Wharton's jelly, (d) prevent compression of the umbilical cord in utero

26. (a) ductus arteriosus, (b) foramen ovale, (c) inferior vena cava, (d) ductus venosus, (e) umbilical vein, (f) umbilical arteries

27. oxygenated, to; deoxygenated, from

28. Fetal circulation differs significantly from infant and adult circulation in that the fetus's oxygenated blood originates from the placenta and flows into the right atrium. It then moves through the foramen ovale (because of the low resistance on the left side of the fetal heart) and out the aorta to provide the head and upper

body with highly oxygenated blood. Very little oxygenated blood flows into the lungs because they are collapsed and offer a high resistance to blood flow. The blood that goes through the pulmonary artery is shunted into the aorta through the ductus arteriosus, bypassing the lungs to supply the rest of the body. See text Chapter 24 for natal circulation.

29. c
30. (a) 16 weeks; (b) 13.5 cm C–R, 15 cm C–H, 200 g; (c) 20 weeks; (d) 4 weeks; (e) 16 weeks; (f) Yes, eyes close at the 10th week and then re-open about the 28th week of gestation.
31. Many factors can influence the development of the embryo or fetus. Significant factors include the quality of the sperm or ova, teratogenic agents such as drugs and radiation, and maternal nutrition. Others you might have identified are any of the complications of pregnancy, such as maternal diabetes, hypertension, or TORCH infections.
32. 8–12
33. (a) Lack of conception despite unprotected sexual intercourse for at least 12 months; (b) Difficulty in conceiving because both partners have decreased fecundity.
34. You could discuss self-care actions that can support fertility, for example avoiding douching and artificial lubricants that alter vaginal pH and adopting positions during intercourse that support retention of sperm. For further self-care measures, see text, Chapter 3.
35. See text, pp. 180–181
36. a
37. d
38. c
39. b
40. g
41. e
42. f
43. See text, pp. 187–188
44. (a) Induces ovulation; dosage range 50–250 mg per day orally, starting day 3 to 5 after menses; can cause hot flushes. (b) A combination of FSH and LH administered IM every day during the first half of the cycle to stimulate follicular development; monitor serum estradiol levels and

ultrasound. (c) Used to treat hyperprolactinemia; side effects may include nausea, diarrhea, dizziness, headaches. (d) Administered via continuous infusion pump; treatment period varies from two to four weeks; may require drugs to augment the various phases of reproductive cycle.

45. a
46. See text, pp. 191–194
47. A possible nursing diagnosis that would apply is *Self-Esteem Disturbance* related to infertility. This diagnosis depends on how successful the couple is in adjusting to the loss of the ability to conceive a child. Other nursing diagnoses that might apply are *Ineffective Individual* (or family) *Coping* related to inability to accept infertility, or *Grieving* related to loss of fertility if the couple has made the decision to accept their childless status.
48. Defining characteristics that are present include negative body image ("... my body can't do what it should"), low self-esteem (expressed feelings of failure), failure in role performance ("I am such a failure as a woman").
49. b
50. karyotype
51. c
52. Each child has a 50-percent chance of developing Huntington's chorea. For diagram, see text, p. 202, Figure 8–15.
53. Because cystic fibrosis is an autosomal recessive disorder, an affected parent must have two genes for the disorder (that is, be homozygous). Thus, with one affected parent and one normal parent, none of the children would have the disorder, but all would be carriers of an abnormal gene for the disorder. See text, p. 202, Figure 8–16.
54. See text, p. 206, Table 8–11.
55. See text, p. 208, Figure 8–20. We hope you have learned interesting and helpful information about your family to facilitate your self-care.
56. (a) amniotic fluid, (b) basal body temperature, (c) human chorionic gonadotropin, (d) human chorionic somatomammotropin, (e) human menopausal gonadotropin, (f) human placental lactogen

# 5 Answer Key

1. Answers may include the following: discontinuing birth control pills at least three months bfore conceiving; strengthening healthful behaviors such as stress reduction, regular exercise, healthy eating; reducing or eliminating behaviors that are known to have adverse affects on pregnancy and fetal growth such as smoking cigarettes/cigars, drinking alcoholic drinks, using illegal drugs. If Max smokes, uses alcohol, or takes illegal drugs, it will be helpful for him to change these behaviors, too.

2. A birth plan is a document formulated by the childbearing couple (or the pregnant woman alone if the father is not involved) that identifies the decisions they have made regarding all aspects of their childbirth experience.

3. Answers may include the following: type of care provider, desired birth setting, participation in prenatal classes, method of childbirth preparation, partner's degree of involvement in the labor and birth, presence of other family members at the birth, use of analgesia/anesthesia, postpartum care, newborn care.

4. See text, p. 221

5. c

6. The uterus, fetus, and placenta require additional blood flow. By the end of pregnancy, one-sixth of the total maternal blood volume is found in the vascular system of the uterus.

7. (a) Chadwick's, (b) Goodell's, (c) Hegar's

8. d

9. Its function is to prevent the ascent of organisms from the vaginal tract into the uterus.

10. stop

11. d

12. Acid pH helps prevent bacterial infections but favors the growth of yeast organisms.

13. (a) increase in size, (b) areolas darken, (c) become more pronounced and enlarged

14. These occur because of estrogen-induced edema and vascular congestion of the nasal mucosa.

15. D

16. I

17. I

18. D

19. I

20. D

21. (a) supine hypotensive, (b) aortocaval, (c) vena caval

22. a

23. (a) The relaxed cardiac sphincter and pressure from the enlarging uterus on the stomach promote reflux of gastric acid secretions into the lower esophagus; (b) Hemorrhoids may be related to constipation and pressure on vessels below the level of the uterus; (c) The pressure of the enlarging uterus in the first and third trimesters increases urinary frequency.

24. b

25. c

26. d

27. b

28. a

29. We are assuming you would take the time to find out if the comments bothered the woman and how she perceives her body image during pregnancy. In answer to her specific questions, you can point out that her "stomach-first walk" occurs because the weight and size of her growing uterus cause her center of gravity to change. To compensate, pregnant women tend to exaggerate the lumbar curve, which may result in backache. Because hormonal effects produce softening of the pelvic joints, the woman's walk assumes a more "waddling" appearance. This may be made more noticeable because many pregnant women also tend to walk with their feet farther apart to help maintain balance.

30. (a) Stimulates estrogen and progesterone production by the corpus luteum until the placenta is sufficiently developed; (b) Stimulates uterine development and development of the ductal

system of the breasts for lactation; (c) Helps maintain pregnancy; also promotes development of the acini and lobules of the breasts for lactation; (d) Decreases maternal metabolism of glucose to favor fetal growth and increases amount of circulating free fatty acids for maternal metabolic needs; (e) Inhibits uterine activity and helps remodel collagen.

31. Prostaglandins may maintain reduced placental vascular resistance. They may also play a role in the initiation of labor.
32. See text, pp. 232–233
33. 25–35 lb (11.5–16 kg)
34. (a) 3.5–5 lb (1.6–2.3 kg); (b) and (c) 12–15 lb (5.5–6.8 kg)
35. S
36. O
37. D
38. S
39. O
40. S
41. O
42. S
43. D
44. O
45. Subjective signs are symptoms the woman experiences and reports; they may have causes other than pregnancy. Objective signs may be perceived by an examiner; they may have causes other than pregnancy. Diagnostic signs are perceived by an examiner and may only be caused by pregnancy.
46. See text, pp. 236–237
47. A positive pregnancy test may be caused by factors other than pregnancy, such as choriocarcinoma, hydatidiform mole, or menopause.
48. c
49. See text, pp. 239–242
50. The effects of pregnancy on a woman's body image are greatly influenced by her feelings about her pregnancy and by cultural, physiologic, psychosocial, and interpersonal factors. Some women experience the "glow of pregnancy" in the second trimester when they begin wearing maternity clothes. In the last weeks of pregnancy, a woman may feel constantly tired and misshapen and may, as a result, have a negative body image.

You are on the right track if you recognized that a variety of factors influence body image. Although there is no one correct answer, certain types of responses occur frequently.

51. Rubin identified the following psychologic tasks of the pregnant woman: (a) Ensuring safe passage through pregnancy, labor, and birth. The woman's concern for herself and her unborn child leads her to select a care giver she trusts and to seek information about birth from classes, friends, and literature. She becomes more concerned about safety—both hers and her partner's. (b) Seeking of acceptance of this child by others. The woman is concerned about her family's acceptance of the child, but her partner's reaction and acceptance are of primary importance to her successful completion of her developmental tasks. She also works to ensure the acceptance of the unborn child by other children in the family. The woman subtly alters her secondary network of friends as necessary to meet the demands of her pregnancy. (c) Seeking of commitment and acceptance of self as mother to the infant—"binding-in." With quickening, the mother begins to develop bonds of attachment to the child and commits herself to the child's welfare. (d) Learning to give of self on behalf of child. The woman begins to develop a capacity for self-denial and delayed personal gratification to meet the needs of another. Baby showers and gifts increase the mother's self-esteem while helping her accept the separateness and needs of her coming child.
52. b
53. We hope you would tell your friend that, even in the most desired pregnancy, feelings of ambivalence are normal. Role changes, physical changes, altered relationships, added financial responsibilities, and attitudes about parenting and values all affect a woman's—indeed a couple's—response to pregnancy.
54. See text, p. 239
55. Traditionally, *couvade* referred to the male's observance of certain rites and rituals as part of his

transition to fatherhood. Today, the term is used to describe the unintentional development of physical symptoms such as fatigue, headache, or difficulty sleeping by the partner of the pregnant woman.

56.  See text, pp. 244–245

57.  It may be difficult initially for a nurse to recognize and accept cultural diversity. To do so, the nurse needs to develop cultural competency. The following points may help a nurse become more effective in caring for people from different cultures: (a) We are all guilty of ethnocentrism occasionally. Ethnocentrism is the belief that one's own cultural beliefs and practices are the best ones. A nurse who finds herself or himself devaluing the practices of another culture should stop and consider that she or he may be demonstrating ethnocentrism. (b) People have a tendency to project their own cultural responses onto people from another culture, and thus they assume that the person is acting from similar motives or values. Often this is not correct and leads to misunderstanding. For example, a nurse who highly values promptness may view a client's lateness as a personal insult when, in reality, the client is much less time-oriented and doesn't place the same value on promptness. (c) Unless there is a clear health contraindication to a particular cultural practice, nurses should avoid interfering in a client's health practices. If the client's beliefs are potentially harmful, the nurse can try to persuade the woman to change. However, if the woman refuses to change, the nurse must accept the woman's right to make her own health choices. (d) Before considering any intervention, the nurse should try to determine the impact of traditional practices on the planned intervention. (e) Practices and beliefs vary not only from one culture to another, but also *within* a culture. These variations are often related to social and economic factors such as class, income, and education. (f) Nurses often find it helpful to begin developing cultural awareness by learning some of the basic beliefs and practices of minority cultures in their area.

If you included some of these ideas, you are well on your way to developing cultural sensitivity. This is a challenging area for health care providers. We hope you can become comfortable working with people from other cultures.

58.  (a) human chorionic gonadotropin, (b) human placental lactogen

# Answer Key

1. d
2. a
3. b
4. f
5. c
6. Alexis is a gravida 4, para 2, ab 1, living children 2.
7. (a) Yolanda is a gravida 3, para 2, ab 0, living children 1. If you recorded this differently, was it because you forgot that a stillborn infant would be considered viable at 36 weeks and would therefore count as a para? (b) Using the detailed approach, Yolanda would be a gravida 3 para 1101. Yolanda's stillborn infant would be considered a preterm birth.
8. Taking an obstetric health history should help you focus on the information that is pertinent to high-quality maternity care. You should be able to identify a reason for each of the questions asked. You should also be able to identify information that may place a client in the high-risk category. In addition to such obvious problems as preexisting medical conditions, think about maternal age, weight, occupation, and previous obstetric history; family history of disorders; marital status and support system; smoking and alcohol consumption; and so on. Once you begin to recognize risk factors, you will be better able to plan for appropriate antepartal care.
9. N
10. A
11. A
12. N
13. N
14. Risk factors are any findings that suggest the pregnancy may have a negative outcome.
15. Answers may include the following: use of addicting drugs; preexisting medical disorders such as diabetes, heart condition, or thyroid disorder; maternal anemia; excessive alcohol consumption; history of habitual spontaneous abortion; multiple gestation; spontaneous premature rupture of the membranes.
16. The initial obstetric examination focuses on inspection, auscultation, and palpation of the abdomen; determination of the adequacy of the pelvis; and vaginal examination.
17. Fundal height is measured in centimeters after the woman has voided. She should lie in the same position each time (generally supine). The zero line of the tape measure is placed on the superior border of the symphysis pubis, and the tape is stretched over the midline of the woman's abdomen to the top of the fundus (see Figure 11–4, p. 269).
18. (a) Between 22–24 weeks and 34 weeks, fundal height in cm generally correlates with weeks of gestation; (b) slightly above the symphysis pubis; (c) at the umbilicus (see Figure 10–6, p. 236).
19. (a) generally by 19–20 weeks' gestation; (b) on average, by 10–12 weeks' gestation.
20. lithotomy
21. The initial pelvic examination should include a Pap smear and any other pertinent cultures or smears; visual inspection of the external genitalia, vagina, and cervix; and a bimanual examination.
22. A diagonal conjugate of 9.0 cm indicates a severely diminished pelvic inlet. In this case, if labor were to occur, the fetal head would probably not be able to enter the pelvic outlet. In spite of uterine contractions, the fetal head would not engage, and the presenting part would probably be described as ballotable, or floating. When a measurement such as this is discovered during the prenatal course, the woman is counseled regarding the need for cesarean birth.
23. Nägele's rule is a method used to determine the estimated date of birth.
24. It is calculated by taking the first day of the LMP, subtracting three months, and adding seven days.

25. Jenny's EDB would be December 29 (± 2 weeks). If you count back February, January, December, it is easy to identify the month. If you set it up as a problem, it is a little more difficult:

| March 22 becomes | 3 – 22 |
| Subtract 3 months | – 3 |
| | 0 – 22 |
| Add 7 days | + 7 |
| EDB | 0 – 29 |

If you remember that January is always the first month, then an answer of "0" becomes December, an answer of "minus 1" would be November, and "minus 2" would be October.

26. Every 4 weeks for first 28 weeks' gestation; every 2 weeks until 36 weeks' gestation, then weekly until childbirth.

27. Answers may include psychologic status, educational needs, support systems, family functioning, economic status, stability of living conditions.

28. c
29. d
30. e
31. a
32. b

33. You should stress to the woman the importance of contacting her care giver immediately if she experiences any of the danger signs in pregnancy.

34. urinary frequency, nausea and vomiting, fatigue, breast tenderness, increased vaginal discharge

35. (a) Wear a well-fitting, supportive bra. (b) Dorsiflex the foot to stretch the affected muscle; apply heat. (c) Eat crackers or dry toast before arising in the morning; have small, frequent meals; avoid causative factors; drink carbonated beverages. (d) Increase fluids, dietary fiber, and exercise. (e) Use proper body mechanics; do pelvic tilt exercise; avoid high-heeled shoes and excessive standing. (f) Void when urge is felt. Increase fluid intake during the day and then decrease fluids *only at night* to decrease nocturia.

36. b

37. *Actions:* In most clinics and offices, laboratory tests are completed at the initial prenatal visit. Thus you could quickly refer to the results of the hemoglobin and hematocrit to determine if Julie is anemic.

*Analysis:* Julie's lab values are within normal limits, so you know she is not anemic. It is tempting at this point to simply assume the fatigue is normal because it is so common among pregnant women. However, this assumption might lead you to miss factors in Julie's life that are contributing to the problem—extra stress at work, the stress of helping a family member with a sick child, or frequent awakenings at night for trips to the bathroom.

*Actions:* An appropriate action might be to provide reassurance while pursuing the matter. You might say, for example, "Many women feel tired during the early months of pregnancy, but sometimes factors or events in the woman's life can add to the fatigue. Is there anything happening in your life that you feel might be contributing to the fatigue?"

*Actions:* Julie's indication that her lifestyle is unchanged suggests that the fatigue is a normal part of her pregnancy. At this point you can begin working with her to plan ways she can get more rest during the day.

38. Begin nipple preparation by going braless occasionally, exposing nipples to air and sunlight; and gently rolling the nipple between the thumb and forefinger for short time each day. Do *not* do rolling exercise if there is a history of preterm labor.

39. Answers may include the following: exercise regularly, at least three times/week; modify exercise intensity based on symptoms; avoid lying supine to exercise after the first trimester; nonweight-bearing exercises such as swimming and cycling are recommended; wear appropriate clothing and supportive shoes; drink plenty of fluids; stop exercising if warning signs such as dizziness, back pain, palpitations, pubic pain, tachycardia, uterine contractions, or vaginal bleeding develop.

40. If you are unsure of the answer, ask your instructor for assistance with this question.

41. Travel by car is fine but can be tiring. She should plan to stop about every two hours and walk around for about 10 minutes. To avoid bladder

trauma she should void regularly. She should wear both lap and shoulder seat belts. The lap belt should be fastened under her abdomen across her upper thighs.

42. Either showers or tub baths are acceptable according to personal preference. Tub baths are contraindicated if there is vaginal bleeding or if the membranes are ruptured because of the risk of introducing infection.

43. (a) early, (b) delayed until after childbirth if possible

44. Although studies do indicate that light drinkers have a risk of complications similar to that of nondrinkers, there is no known safe level of alcohol consumption during pregnancy and women are best advised to abstain from all alcohol.

45. A possible nursing diagnosis would be ***Knowledge Deficit*** related to lack of information about guidelines for sexual activity during the third trimester. Perhaps you chose ***Sexual Dysfunction*** related to lack of knowledge. It is tempting because the problem concerns sexual activity, and some people would support this diagnosis. However, because their sexual activity is satisfying to both and they have adapted their practices in light of the pregnancy, they do not meet the definition of a dysfunction. They are simply seeking information.

46. teratogen

47. Answers may include the following: women who delay childbirth tend to be well educated and financially secure; they tend to be emotionally stable; their pregnancies are usually planned, and the baby is wanted; they typically obtain early prenatal care; they are more aware of the realities of having a child.

48. c

49. Answers may include the following: concerns about ability to parent well; about whether they have sufficient energy to care for a baby; about their ability to deal with an older child as they age; about the financial impact of having a college-age child as they near retirement; about the social isolation they feel as older parents.

50. Answers may include the following: needing someone to love; unstable family relationships; competition with mother; desire to punish parent(s); desire for emancipation from home; cultural values that support early pregnancy; unmotivated accident; lack of understanding about contraceptive options, incest, feelings of love for partner.

51. This question gives you a lot of room to plan creatively. Obviously, there is no one right answer. We hope that in planning your clinic you keep in mind that the early adolescent is often quite different in needs and interaction from the late adolescent. Although the older adolescent can often think abstractly, many adolescents are very concrete thinkers and tend to be present-oriented and egocentric. Thus it is helpful to use audiovisual aids and provide "hands-on" learning experiences. Activities have more meaning if the adolescent sees them as having a specific value for her.

In planning, we hope you emphasize a multi-disciplinary approach that also includes the father of the child and the parents of the adolescent mother and father (if the adolescents wish them to be involved). This leads to the question of choice: It is important to give these adolescents choices and to help them learn to make appropriate decisions. Thus some guidance may be beneficial, but too much may keep them from learning how to make choices and decisions.

Finally, we hope you give some thought to the atmosphere of your clinic: Is it open, non-judgmental, and supportive? Do the adolescents feel free to ask questions and express fears? Does it feel safe and free of coercion?

52. c

53. See text, pp. 326–327

54. Ideal weight gain during pregnancy for a woman of normal weight is a gain of 3.5–5 lb (1.6–2.3 kg) during the first trimester, followed by a gain of about 1 lb (0.4–0.5 kg) per week during the second and third trimesters.

55. 300

56. a

57. a

58. i

59. b

60.  c
61.  d
62.  e
63.  h
64.  f
65.  g
66.  Pregnant vegetarians often use soybean products such as soybean milk, tofu, and soy protein isolates as a source of protein. Other sources include nuts and lentils. Possible additional sources of calcium include turnip greens, white beans, and almonds.

67.  This woman's diet had 4 servings of grain products. This is adequate. She had 4 servings of protein, which is more than adequate. However, since she only had 2½ servings of dairy products (recommended is 4) and 3 fruits or vegetables (4–6 are recommended), her diet is deficient in these areas.

68.  (a) estimated date of birth, (b) estimated date of confinement, (c) estimated date of delivery, (d) fetal activity diary, (e) fetal movement record, (f) gravida, (g) para, (h) recommended dietary allowance

# 7 Answer Key

1. Fetal alcohol syndrome
2. IUGR, altered brain development, malformations of the genitourinary tract, irritability, increased risk of SIDS
3. IUGR, meconium aspiration, hypoxia, addiction
4. One; ten
5. Answers may include the following: general health status, nutritional status, risk of infection, all body systems, woman's knowledge of the impact of substance abuse on her or her fetus.
6. Preferred methods include psychoprophylaxis, regional analgesia/anesthesia such as an epidural or local anesthesia.
7. False. Although there is a tendency to assume that administering an analgesic to a woman who is a substance abuser will increase her addiction, this assumption is not correct. The woman should receive the support necessary to help her deal effectively with the discomfort of labor and birth.
8. Answers include polyuria, polyphagia, polydipsia, weight loss.
9. c
10. d
11. Answers may include changes in insulin requirements; decreased renal threshold for glucose; increased risk of ketoacidosis, insulin shock, and coma; possible acceleration of vascular disease.
12. Answers may include hydramnios, maternal ketoacidosis, fetal death, increased incidence of fetal anomalies, macrosomia, birth trauma, asphyxia.
13. Belle Lee did maintain effective control. Glycosylated hemoglobin is an accurate indicator of a person's long-term control. In the presence of elevated blood glucose levels, hemoglobin $A_0$ converts to hemoglobin $A_{1c}$ or glycosylated hemoglobin. Since the process is essentially irreversible, elevations indicate that the person has been hyperglycemic. The normal range is approximately 6 percent to 8 percent. Thus, Ms Lee's glycohemoglobin level of 7.0 percent is within normal limits.
14. Your intervention was very effective. You began by asking Ms Lee for her opinion about ways of helping her keep her appointment. As is often the case, the client herself had obviously thought about the problem and tried to correct it but was unable to do so without assistance. By working in a collaborative way with Ms Lee and the physician, you were able to arrange an effective solution. Good job!
15. Two injections of insulin spread out over the day results in more stable blood sugar levels because the types of insulin used—generally regular and NPH—peak at different times.
16. She should exercise after meals when blood sugar levels are high; she should wear diabetic identification and should carry hard candy for a rapid source of sugar. In addition, she should monitor her blood glucose regularly and avoid injecting insulin into an extremity that will soon be used during exercise.
17. a
18. Oral hypoglycemic agents are used in treating certain types of diabetes. However, because they have been linked to fetal abnormalities, they are contraindicated during pregnancy.
19. Infants who are large at birth generally have mothers who are class A, B, or C diabetics. The infants are exposed to high glucose levels in utero. In response, the fetus produces high levels of insulin and uses the available glucose. This increased use leads to excessive growth (macrosomia).
20. Answers may include maternal serum $\alpha$-fetoprotein, ultrasound, fetal biophysical profile, nonstress tests, contraction stress test.
21. (a) Insufficient hemoglobin production related to nutritional deficiency of iron or folic acid;

(b) hemoglobin destruction in an inherited disorder such as sickle cell anemia or thalassemia.

22. Iron deficiency anemia
23. See text, p. 368
24. (a) 17, (b) zidovudine
25. Answers may include weight loss, fever, oral infections such as thrush, pneumonia, lymph node enlargement, enlarged liver and spleen.
26. Gloves should be worn when contact with blood, body fluids, nonintact skin, or mucous membranes is possible.
27. d
28. a
29. (a) Asymptomatic. No limitation of physical activity. (b) Slight limitation of physical activity. Asymptomatic at rest; symptoms occur with heavy physical activity. (c) Moderate to marked limitation of physical activity. Symptoms occur during less-than-ordinary physical activity. (d) Inability to carry out any physical activity without discomfort. Even at rest the person experiences symptoms of cardiac insufficiency or anginal pain.

30. Answers may include cough, dyspnea, edema, heart murmurs, palpitations, rales, weight gain.
31. b
32. b
33. Penicillin is started as prophylaxis to prevent recurrent bouts of rheumatic fever and subsequent heart valve damage.
34. Whenever possible, vaginal birth is preferred, using low forceps and a local or regional anesthetic to decrease the stress of the second stage of labor. This procedure also avoids the hazards associated with abdominal surgery for cesarean birth.
35. (a) acquired immunodeficiency syndrome, (b) diabetes mellitus, (c) fetal alcohol syndrome, (d) gestational diabetes mellitus, (e) human immunodeficiency virus, (f) insulin-dependent diabetes mellitus

# Answer Key

1. The goals of therapy are to control vomiting, correct dehydration, restore electrolyte balance, and maintain adequate nutrition.
2. b
3. e
4. d
5. f
6. c
7. a
8. See text, pp. 388–389
9. A D&C is performed to remove the remainder of the products of conception.
10. Answers may include chromosomal abnormalities, teratogenic drugs, placental abnormalities, faulty implantation, chronic maternal disease, maternal infection, endocrine imbalances.
11. Answers may include cervical trauma, congenital cervical structural defects, uterine anomalies.
12. Shirodkar-Barter operation (cerclage)
13. Implantation of the blastocyst in a site other than the endometrial lining of the uterus.
14. fallopian tubes
15. See text, pp. 390–391
16. c
17. d
18. Continued high or rising hCG levels are abnormal and may indicate the development of choriocarcinoma. Periodic examinations are necessary to detect rising levels. Ms Chan should avoid pregnancy because otherwise it would be difficult to tell whether elevated hCG levels were related to pregnancy or developing malignancy.
19. Rupture of the membranes before 37 weeks' gestation.
20. Respiratory distress syndrome (RDS)
21. Infection
22. Nitrazine paper; blue or blue-green; alkaline
23. Answers may include continue on bed rest with bathroom privileges; monitor temperature four times daily; avoid sexual intercourse, douches, and tampons; contact physician if she has fever, uterine tenderness, contractions, increased leakage of fluid, decreased fetal movement, foul-smelling vaginal discharge.
24. Previous preterm birth, smoking 15 cigarettes a day, history of pyelonephritis, bleeding at 14 weeks' gestation, low socioeconomic level.
25. To answer Mrs Smythe, you will need to include the following: She will need to watch for signs of preterm labor, which include uterine contractions every 10 minutes or less, mild menstrual-like cramps felt low in the abdomen, feelings of pelvic pressure, low backache that is constant or comes and goes, a change in vaginal discharge, and abdominal cramping with or without diarrhea.

    Teach her to lie down on her side or tilted to one side with a pillow. She may then place her fingertips on the fundus of the uterus. She checks for contractions (hardening or tightening) for about 1 hour. If contractions are felt every 10 minutes for 1 hour, she needs to call her health care provider.
26. A contraction will feel like a hardening or tightening of the uterus. She may also note a backache that comes and goes on a regular pattern of every 10 minutes. This may be associated with contractions.
27. Y
28. Y
29. N
30. N
31. N
32. Y
33. Y
34. N
35. Magnesium sulfate decreases the frequency and intensity of uterine contractions.
36. (a) 4–6, (b) 2–4
37. calcium
38. See text, p. 402

39. Helen Polawski has a number of factors present that contraindicate beginning therapy to stop her labor. She is 5 cm dilated, and her contractions indicate active labor. Her membranes have been ruptured for just short of 24 hours, and although you do not know the cause of her low-grade fever, you should suspect amnionitis at this point.

    These factors would lead you to answer "no." The most pressing nursing goal is probably to prepare her for childbirth. With three previous births, a small baby this time (34 weeks' gestation), and 5 cm dilatation with active labor, the birth may be just a few minutes away.

40. (a) 3, (b) 4, (c) NA, (d) 2, (e) 1, (f) NA, (g) NA

41. *Actions:* We hope you would check Ms George's blood pressure and test her urine for protein.
    *Analysis:* Ms George's BP is elevated significantly. An increase of 30/15 indicates mild preeclampsia. Ms George's BP has increased 42/26, her urine contains protein, and she has had a major weight gain. Her symptoms indicate more than mild preeclampsia. We hope that at this point you would assess Rita for further signs of severe preeclampsia.
    *Assessments:* At this point you could ask Ms George about additional symptoms such as headache, visual changes, or epigastric pain. You can quickly assess deep tendon reflexes and observe for evidence of edema.
    *Actions:* You now have a clear picture of Ms George's status and should report your findings to the physician. Your preliminary assessments will help the physician realize the need to see Ms George quickly. Since you would expect the physician to admit Ms George to the hospital, you can quickly confirm his or her intentions and begin the necessary procedures for admission. You will thus avoid unnecessary delays for Ms George.
    *Analysis:* You know that the unexpected hospitalization must be stressful for Ms George. You also realize that she must have many questions and concerns.
    *Actions:* Take the time to explain things to Ms George and answer her questions. She will probably be worried about the impact of the PIH on her unborn child and may also be worried about the problems caused for her family by her hospitalization. Having an opportunity to talk, plan, and consider her alternatives will be especially helpful. You can also offer to contact Ms George's family and explain the situation. If she is upset, it may be necessary to arrange with them to transport her to the hospital. Any support and assistance you can provide will be very helpful to her.

42. See text, pp. 410–411

43. Grand mal seizures or coma

44. c

45. See text, p. 412

46. d

47. (a) 6, (b) 15–20, (c) 2

48. Answers include diminished or absent reflexes, depressed respirations, marked lethargy.

49. *h*emolysis, *e*levated *l*iver enzymes, *l*ow *p*latelet count

50. 3+ DTRs are brisker than average but may not be abnormal.

51. To assess for clonus, the nurse quickly dorsiflexes the woman's foot. When there is hyperreflexia, the foot will jerk. Each movement (jerk) is counted, so two beats of clonus means there were two movements after the foot was dorsiflexed.

52. If you answered "no," you were right on target. Carolyn Lorenzo is not a candidate for RhoGAM because her indirect Coombs' test indicates that she has already been sensitized to Rh+ blood and has developed antibodies. Since her first baby was Rh–, it is not known when Carolyn became sensitized. She may have had an undiagnosed pregnancy that ended in early miscarriage, she may have had a blood transfusion with Rh+ blood, or she may have had a small placental bleed during this pregnancy. Regardless of when it occurred, she needs a clear explanation of the risks she faces for hemolytic disease in subsequent pregnancies and her newborn needs to be evaluated carefully.

53. It provides passive antibody protection against Rh antigens.

54. See text, pp. 426–427

55. a

56. b
57. first
58. d
59. a
60. c
61. b
62. We hope you would tell her that, while there is a lower incidence of herpes infection in infants born by cesarean, cesarean birth is not guaranteed to prevent herpes infection in the newborn. Moreover, it does carry the risk of surgery for the mother. Currently, the recommended approach to deciding about the route of birth is to examine the woman carefully for signs of lesions and ask her about the presence of any prodromal symptoms. If either is present, cesarean birth is indicated. If no signs of infection are present, the woman will probably give birth vaginally. The woman may also find it helpful to talk with her care giver about taking an oral antiviral medication such as acyclovir (Zovirax), beginning several weeks before her anticipated due date in order to suppress the infection.

63. (a) cytomegalic inclusion disease; (b) cytomegalovirus; (c) disseminated intravascular coagulation; (d) deep tendon reflexes; (e) pregnancy-induced hypertension; (f) sexually transmitted disease; (g) sexually transmitted infection; (h) TO toxoplasmosis, R rubella, C cytomegalovirus, H herpes virus II

# 9 Answer Key

1. Some advantages of ultrasound testing include the following: transabdominal method is non-invasive, it is a generally painless procedure with the exception of discomfort from a full bladder (for ultrasound in the first two trimesters), it allows for differentiation of soft tissues, immediate information may be gained.

2. Early pregnancy uses include ability to determine gestational sac and placement of the sac, identification of the embryo or fetus, number of embryos or fetuses, presence or absence of fetal heart activity, fetal measurements for growth, location of the placenta. Late pregnancy uses include following fetal growth patterns, locating the placenta, validating fetal presentation and position, investigating congenital anomalies or problems, assessing amount of amniotic fluid, completing a biophysical profile, locating the umbilical cord for cordocentesis.

3. There are no known ill effects from ultrasound to date. Ultrasound has been in use for more than 30 years.

4. At this time, Hazel's uterus is lower than expected and she should have felt fetal movement. Ultrasound can provide information regarding the gestation.

5. Explain that she will have to drink water to fill her bladder; then an abdominal or vaginal ultrasound probe will be used. The test should not be uncomfortable.

6. (a) Your teaching plan should include the following points: begin assessing at about 30–32 weeks; during rest periods, gently place her hand on the fundus to detect fetal movement and to feel uterine contractions. See text for further information. (b) Her attentiveness during each assessment period will be important. The fetus tends to move more after the mother has eaten. It is important that the mother understand the fetus has periods of sleep, during which fetal movement may not be felt for 20–40 minutes.

7. To determine fetal well-being, measured by the ability of the fetus to respond to its body movement with an acceleration of the FHR.

8. See text, Chapter 17

9. See text, Chapter 17

10. Reactive NST. This test demonstrates that the fetus is able to respond to movement with an acceleration of the FHR. The fetus is not stressed and has reserve to cope with changes in the environment.

11. Figure 9–1A is reactive. Figure 9–1B is nonreactive.

12. Fetal acoustic stimulation may be used when the NST is nonreactive. A sound is transmitted through the maternal abdomen into the uterus. A fetus who is asleep will respond to the sound with an acceleration in FHR. If the fetus is stressed and unable to respond, the NST will remain nonreactive and further assessment is needed immediately.

13. (a) The five biophysical variables are fetal breathing movements, gross body movements, fetal tone, reactive fetal heart rate, qualitative amniotic fluid volume. (b) Each biophysical variable is scored as 2 or 0. A "good" score is 10 (2 points on each variable) or 8 (as long as amniotic fluid volume received a score of 2). (c) In any situation in which the fetus is thought to be at risk due to maternal or fetal factors. (d) Decreased amniotic fluid is associated with oligohydramnios. The fetus is at increased risk because the umbilical cord does not have enough fluid to float in and may become compressed. (e) Your teaching plan should include what the test is; the anticipated usefulness, benefits, risks, and interpretations of the results; and whom to contact for further information.

14. Maternal indications for a CST include diabetes mellitus, heart disease, preeclampsia, suspected postmaturity, history of previous stillborn, Rh sensitization, abnormal estriol excretion, hyperthyroidism, and kidney disease. Fetal

indications include IUGR and nonreactive NST.

15. Contraindications include third trimester bleeding, previous cesarean birth with classic uterine incision, presence of placenta previa.

16. See text, Chapter 17

17. A BBST involves stimulating endogenous oxytocin. A CST depends on IV administration of oxytocin (exogenous).

18. a

19. b

20. (a) The CST tracing is negative. (b) There are no late decelerations with uterine contractions. Note: Three contractions have occurred in just over 8 minutes.

21. Draw any of the test results. Visualization of results helps you learn.

22. Amniocentesis provides a specimen of amniotic fluid for testing.

23. Ultrasound guidance is essential.

24. Nursing interventions during an amniocentesis should include the following: prepare the equipment, cleanse the abdomen, assess the maternal vital signs and the FHR prior to amniocentesis and after the procedure is completed, document amniocentesis in the client's chart, provide information and support to the client.

25. Complications may include infection (from contamination of the uterine contents with pathogens), continued leakage of amniotic fluid (from failure of the puncture site to close), bleeding (from puncture of the placenta or umbilical cord), irritation of the uterus that results in contractions (treated with a betasympathomimetic).

26. The L/S ratio test determines the amount of lecithin to sphingomyelin. Normal results are 2:1 and indicate that the fetus has sufficient surfactant to support extrauterine respirations. The phosphatidyglycerol test determines the presence or absence of another key phospholipid in surfactant. The presence of phosphatidylglycerol also indicates that adequate amounts of surfactant are present. Creatinine is a nondirect estimation of fetal age. The test is based on the knowledge that most fetuses of 34–36 weeks' gestation have a body weight that results in excretion of 2 mL/100 mL of amniotic fluid. Findings of 2 mL/100 mL of amniotic fluid provide information that the fetus is probably of 34–36 weeks' gestation. This particular test is unreliable when the fetus is not of expected weight.

27. *Actions:* You need to know more about the contraction characteristics (such as frequency, duration, and intensity of contractions) and whether there are any additional signs of labor.
    *Actions:* You will need to reiterate the discharge instructions, which should include signs of labor, how to assess uterine contractions, and signs of infections.

28. The correct answer is yes. The L/S ratio is mature, and the presence of PG is also associated with fetal lung maturity.

29. (a) amniotic fluid volume, (b) breast self-stimulation test, (c) biophysical profile, (d) crown-rump length, (e) contraction stress test, (f) fetal acoustical stimulation test, (g) fetal body movement, (h) femur length, (i) head circumference, (j) intrauterine growth retardation, (k) lecithin-sphingomyelin ratio, (l) nipple stimulation contraction stress test, (m) nonstress test, (n) phosphatidylglycerol, (o) ultrasound, (p) vibratory stimulation test

# 10 Answer Key

1. The inlet and pelvic cavity of the gynecoid pelvis are rounded; therefore, all the pelvic diameters are more likely to be adequate for the fetus to pass through during labor and birth. The anthropoid pelvis tends to be more heart-shaped but still provides adequate measurements for the fetus to pass through.

2. The android (typical male pelvis) is wide from front to back but very narrow from side to side. This interferes with descent of the fetus into the inlet. The platypelloid pelvic inlet is very wide from side to side so descent of the fetal head into the pelvis is more likely than with an android; however, the inlet is very narrow front to back and this interferes with internal rotation.

3. See text, Chapter 18

4. b

5. d

6. (a) occipital bone, (b) lambdoidal suture, (c) posterior fontanelle, (d) sagittal suture, (e) parietal bone, (f) coronal suture, (g) anterior fontanelle, (h) mitotic suture

7. The sutures of the fetal skull are membranous spaces between the cranial bones. The intersections of the sutures are called fontanelles.

8. c

9. d

10. b

11. a

12. The anterior and posterior fontanelles are the intersections between the sutures. The anterior fontanelle allows growth of the brain by remaining unossified for as long as 18 months. The posterior fontanelle closes between 8–12 weeks after birth. During labor and birth, the descent and position of the fetal head can be assessed by palpating the posterior suture.

13. (a) The anterior fontanelle is located between the coronal, frontal, and sagittal suture and is diamond shaped. (b) The posterior fontanelle is located between the sagittal and the lambdoidal suture and is triangular in shape.

14. (a) anterior fontanelle, (b) vertex, (c) posterior fontanelle, (d) occiput, (e) mastoid fontanelle, (f) mentum (chin), (g) sphenoid fontanelle, (h) sinciput (brow)

15. *View A.* (a) suboccipitobregmatic, (b) 9.5 cm, (c) occipitofrontal, (d) 11.75 cm, (e) occipitomental, (f) 13.5 cm. *View B.* (g) biparietal diameter, (h) 9.25 cm, (i) bitemporal diameter, (j) 8 cm

16. c

17. a

18. b

19. See text, p. 475

20. The fetal presentation is determined by fetal lie and by the body part of the fetus that enters the mother's pelvis first.

21. vertex, military, brow, face

22. Complete breech (fetal buttocks down against cervix), frank breech (fetal buttocks down against cervix, fetal legs up against abdomen and chest), footling (one or both feet are against the cervix).

23. (a) cephalic presentation, (b) ROA, (c) presenting part–occiput

24. (a) cephalic presentation, (b)LOP, (c) presenting part–occiput

25. (a) cephalic presentation, (b) LOA, (c) presenting part–occiput

26. (a) cephalic presentation, (b) LOT, (c) presenting part–occiput

27. (a) cephalic presentation, (b) ROP, (c) presenting part–occiput

28. (a) breech presentation, (b) LSA, (c) presenting part–sacrum

29. (a) breech presentation, (b) RSA, (c) presenting part–sacrum

30. (a) cephalic (face) presentation, (b) LMA, (c) presenting part–mentum

31. (a) cephalic (face) presentation, (b) RMP, (c) presenting part–mentum

32. (a) breech presentation, (b) LSP, (c) presenting part–sacrum

33. (a) transverse lie, (b) LAPA, (c) presenting part–shoulder

34. (a) cephalic (face) presentation, (b) RMA, (c) presenting part–mentum

35. (a) breech presentation, (b) single footling, (c) presenting part–single footling

    If you had difficulty with this question, refer back to the definitions of presentation and position. It may also help to use a model of a pelvis with a fetus. This is an important aspect, so keep at it.

36. Methods include Leopold's maneuvers, visual inspection of the maternal abdomen, location of fetal heart rate, vaginal examination, assessment of the mother's greatest area of discomfort (posterior position is associated with severe backache), visualization by ultrasound.

37. Engagement of the presenting part occurs when the largest diameter of the presenting part reaches or passes through the pelvic inlet.

38. None. Engagement provides information about the inlet but not about the midpelvis or outlet. Fetal descent would provide information about the midpelvis and outlet.

39. Leopold's maneuvers and vaginal examinations can be used to determine engagement.

40. Questions such as the following should be directed toward changes the mother might feel once engagement has occurred. (a) "Have you recently noticed a change in the way your clothes fit?" Rationale: As the fetal head drops into the inlet, there may be a change in the shape of the abdomen. It may seem that the baby has dropped down and away from the mother's body. This causes a change in the way her clothes fit. (b) "Have you recently noticed that you have to urinate more frequently?" Rationale: As the fetus descends into the pelvis, there may be more pressure on the bladder. (c) "Have you noticed more discomfort in your pelvic area and your thighs?" Rationale: As the fetus descends into the pelvis, there may be more discomfort. There may also be increased pressure from vasocongestion of the areas below the pelvis (that is, the perineum and the lower extremities). (d) "Have you noticed easier breathing?" Rationale: As the fetus descends into the pelvis, there may be less pressure on the diaphragm.

    Any of these changes may suggest that engagement has occurred, but they are not diagnostic.

41. *Station* refers to the relationship of the presenting part to an imaginary line drawn between the ischial spines of the maternal pelvis.

42. Minus (–) 1 station means the presenting part is 1 cm above the ischial spines.

43. Failure to descend may be associated with cephalopelvic disproportion, malposition, malpresentation, asynclitism, multiple pregnancy.

44. c

45. b

46. e

47. d

48. a

49. f

50. (a) increment, (b) acme, (c) decrement, (d) duration, (e) frequency

51. Factors may include expectant mother's desire for this baby, amount of education (general and childbirth), coping skills, support from others, worry about the pregnancy or about being a parent, view of self, role changes, worry about finances, fear that she will not be able to tolerate the labor and birth in the way she wishes, association of pregnancy, labor and/or birth with previous abuse.

52. Culture shapes our worldview and our ideas about role, behavior, customs, the way we respond to challenges or pain, what we want for comfort, eating and drinking preferences, and so on.

53. c

54. c

55. d

56. *First:* from beginning of true labor to complete dilatation. *Second:* from complete dilatation to birth of baby. *Third:* from birth of baby to birth of placenta. *Fourth:* from birth of placenta to 2–4 hours after birth.

57.  (a) latent, (b) active, (c) transitional
58.  first stage, latent phase
59.  (a) 1.2 cm/hr, (b) 1.5 cm/hr for a multigravida
60.  Frequency every 2–2.5 minutes, duration 60–75 seconds, intensity strong.
61.  Physiologic causes of pain during labor are uterine muscle hypoxia as contractions occur and become longer, closer, and stronger; stretching of the cervix as it dilates and effaces; pressure of the presenting part on the cervix; stretching of the vaginal and perineal tissues; exhaustion.
62.  Key factors include psychosocial-cultural factors such as age, maturity level, educational level, amount of knowledge regarding childbirth, availability of supportive person, coping abilities, ability to make decisions and make wishes known, cultural expectations and opportunities for expressions of pain, fear, and anxiety.
63.  (a) left-acromion-dorsal-anterior, (b) left-acromion-dorsal-posterior, (c) left-mentum-anterior, (d) left-mentum-posterior, (e) left-mentum-transverse, (f) left-occiput-anterior, (g) left-occiput-posterior, (h) left-occiput-transverse, (i) left-sacrum-anterior, (j) left-sacrum-posterior, (k) left-sacrum-transverse, (l) right-mentum-anterior, (m) right-mentum-posterior, (n) right-mentum-transverse, (o) right-occiput-anterior, (p) rupture of membranes, (q) right-occiput-posterior, (r) right-occiput-transverse, (s) right-sacrum-anterior, (t) right-sacrum-posterior, (u) right-sacrum-transverse

# 11  Answer Key

1. The answers will depend on the role your friend takes. Answer all the questions you can. Practice different ways of phrasing questions so that you are best able to elicit answers to the questions.

2. (a) Culture shapes our beliefs, values, and expectations of each event in our life. You have your own beliefs about touch, method of communication, how close you want someone when you are talking, whether you look at the person talking to you, whether you express your discomfort when you are having pain or whether you are quiet, and who may be with you. Other cultures may differ from what you want or expect.

   (b) The most important action is to honor the family's beliefs and needs if at all possible. Most birthing centers or hospitals have male or female lab techs available. Outside the client's room, explain to the laboratory technician that the family's cultural beliefs prohibit a male from performing any care and that you will need to call for a female tech.

3. There are four pertinent assessments of uterine contractions: intensity, frequency, duration, and the client's response to the contractions.

4. Fingertips are more sensitive and provide less pressure.

5. Contraction frequency of 10–20 minutes, duration 15–20 seconds, mild intensity; progressing to frequency of 5–7 minutes, duration 30–40 seconds, moderate intensity.

6. (a) every 5 min, (b) 30 sec, (c) mild

7. 

| Contraction Begins | Contraction Ends |
|---|---|
| 0500:00 | 0500:40 |
| | (duration 40 seconds) |
| 0505:00 | 0505:40 |
| (frequency 5 min) | (duration 40 seconds) |
| 0508:00 | 0508:45 |
| (frequency 3 min) | (duration 45 seconds) |

| Contraction Begins | Contraction Ends |
|---|---|
| 0511:00 | 0511:45 |
| (frequency 3 min) | (duration 45 seconds) |

   Remember, frequency is the time from the beginning of one contraction to the beginning of the next contraction. (a) The frequency indicated by the first two contractions is 5 minutes; the frequency from the second through the fourth contraction is 3 minutes. This would be recorded as every 3–5 minutes. (b) The duration is 40–45 seconds.

8. Mild feels like a slightly contracted biceps muscle. Moderate is similar to a tightly contracted biceps muscle. Strong is similar to feeling the back of your hand: it cannot be indented by your fingers.

9. (a) Locate the FHR by beginning in the lower left segment of the maternal uterus and then work in ever-enlarging circles until the FHR is heard. (b) You check the maternal pulse and listen to the FHR to make sure that the rates are different. The FHR should be more rapid than that of the normal laboring woman. (c) It is best to listen for at least 30 seconds, and every so often you should listen for 60 seconds. During the labor, it is important to listen through a contraction to detect any slowing of the heart rate if an electronic fetal monitor is not being used. Guidelines for when to listen in low-risk situations are as follows: every 30 minutes during the first stage (active and transition phase), every 15 minutes during the second stage. It is important to listen to FHR immediately after the rupture of amniotic membranes, if the amniotic fluid has a greenish color (meconium staining); after an enema if given; after any analgesic or regional block; and with any significant change of maternal vital signs or change in fetal activity.

10. The woman should be lying on her back with a small pillow under her head. The knees are

drawn up, with feet flat on the bed to increase relaxation of the abdominal muscles.

11. (a) cephalic, (b) right occiput. Note that you were not given enough specific information to determine whether the right (R) occiput (O) was anterior (ROA) or posterior (ROP). Think through what your hands would feel if the fetus was LOA, LOP, or RSA (right-sacrum-anterior).

12. The membrane status is ascertained beforehand because the lubricant used for the vaginal examination can change the reactivity of the Nitrazine test tape and thereby give a false reading.

13. Intact membranes act as a dilating wedge against the cervix and protect the fetal head from compression against the cervix.

14. Ruptured membranes (ROM) allow for greater pressure to be applied to the cervix during contractions by the fetal head and therefore may hasten cervical dilatation and effacement. Once membranes are ruptured, there is an open pathway into the uterus and infection may occur in the uterine cavity if ROM is prolonged.

15. Most sources recommend that the birth occur within 24 hours after rupture of membranes because after that time the incidence of infection increases. You will need to know when they rupture to be able to keep track of the 24 hours.

16. When membranes rupture, the umbilical cord may prolapse (umbilical cord may be washed down ahead of the fetal head into the cervix or vagina). This will most likely be indicated by a decrease in the FHR.

17. To assist Joelle, consider the following: you need to assess her information base and understanding of the benefits and risks of amniotomy. Provide additional information as needed. Make sure she understands the risks and benefits and has an opportunity to talk further with her certified nurse-midwife or physician.

18. Your response might be something like: "Mrs X would prefer not to have an amniotomy done."

19. You might say, "Mrs. X has said she would prefer not to have an amniotomy. Is there something you are finding that she needs to know to reconsider her decision?" You are in a position to continue to be the client advocate. As you ask further questions, be direct and work to facilitate the exchange of information between Mrs X and her physician.

20. (a) The membranes are intact. The Nitrazine test is negative. (b) The most likely source of the clear fluid is the bladder.

21. (a) A number of assessments are made while performing a vaginal examination. You can determine cervical effacement and dilatation; determine fetal descent, station, position, and presentation; and assess pelvic measurements. (b) Position her in low-Fowler's with her heels together and knees out to the side. Use the sheet or a warm blanket to drape her legs and vulva. Make sure the door to the room is closed and the curtains around the bed are closed.

22. (a) 3 cm. If you did not answer this correctly, refer to appendix on cervical dilatations in your textbook. (b) Cephalic. The head feels firm compared to the softer tissues of its buttocks when the fetus is in a breech presentation. (c) Left occiput anterior (LOA). The triangular shape is the posterior fontanelle. If it is felt in the upper portion of the cervix, the fetus is LOA. Refer to Figure 10–5c (or your textbook) for help in visualizing this fetal position. (d) Rupture of capillaries in the cervix.

23. (a) Describe what a "miniprep" is, the information regarding advantages and disadvantages, and any possible side effects. (b) Three effects of an enema are to cleanse the lower bowel, to stimulate uterine contractions, and to avoid client embarrassment during the second stage of labor. (c) If her membranes have ruptured, she should expel the enema into a bedpan. Consider leaving the side rails up to provide something for her to hold on to. If her labor is advancing rapidly, you will need to assess her labor status frequently. And when she is expelling an enema in the bathroom, she will need to know how to call for assistance.

24. Aspects of the Lamaze breathing are presented in the text on page 558.

25. You can provide Henri with information and opportunities for questions. He can support Joelle with comfort measures such as fluids, a comfortable place to sit, and encouragement and support.

26. Fetal baseline refers to the average FHR obtained during a 10-minute period of monitoring. Fetal tachycardia is a sustained rate of 160 beats/min or above. Fetal bradycardia is a rate less than 120 beats/min. Baseline variability is called short-term or long-term. Short-term is the beat-to-beat change in the heart rate, and long-term is the waviness or rhythmic fluctuations of the FHR tracing. Deceleration is the periodic decrease in FHR from the normal baseline. For definitions of early, late, and variable deceleration, see the answer to question 31 below.

27. (a) electronic fetal monitor, (b) fetal heart rate, (c) uterine activity, (d) uteroplacental insufficiency, (e) head compression, (f) cord compression

28. (a) 120, (b) 160, (c) present, (d) average, (e) no

29. The possible causes of fetal tachycardia include prematurity, mild or chronic fetal hypoxia, fetal infection, frequent repetitive fetal movements, maternal anxiety, maternal drugs, high maternal temperature, fetal arrhythmias.

30. The possible causes of fetal bradycardia include fetal hypoxia; sudden hypoxemia; arrhythmia, such as congenital heart block; hypothermia; drugs, such as beta-adrenergic blocking agents (anesthetic agent used for paracervical block).

31. The possible causes of changes in baseline variability include maternal medications, fetal rest, gestation of less than 32 weeks, fetal hypoxia and acidosis, fetal malformation.

32. (a) Early deceleration occurs when the fetal head is compressed and cerebral blood flow is decreased, which leads to central vagal stimulation and results in a slowing of the FHR. (b) Late deceleration is caused by uteroplacental insufficiency resulting from decreased blood flow and oxygen transfer to the fetus through the intervillous spaces during uterine contractions. (c) Variable deceleration occurs if the umbilical cord becomes compressed.

33. (a) every 1.5 to 2 minutes, (b) 40–60 seconds. Early decelerations.

34. Contraction frequency: 1 min to 1 min 40 seconds; duration: 40–80 seconds. Type of FHR pattern: late decelerations. Variability: average.

Contraction frequency is *not* within normal expectations. Contractions should not exceed a frequency of every 2 minutes nor a duration of more than 75 (or at most 90) seconds.

35. Contraction frequency: every 2 minutes; duration: 50–60 seconds. Type of FHR pattern: variable decelerations.

36. Late decelerations: Since late decelerations are caused by uteroplacental insufficiency, all nursing actions should be directed toward increasing perfusion to the placenta and fetus. Interventions would include turning the laboring woman to her side (left or right); checking maternal BP for hypotension and either increasing IV flow rate (with physiologic fluid) or beginning an IV if hypotension is present; starting oxygen per face mask; and of course, immediately reassessing for expected improvement as a result of the interventions and notifying the certified nurse-midwife or physician. Variable decelerations are caused by compression on the fetal umbilical cord. Nursing actions would be focused on relieving the cord compression by changing the woman's position.

37. (a) The client history should indicate no use of narcotics because Stadol will precipitate a withdrawal. Maternal knowledge base regarding the medication, maternal BP, and FHR status should be assessed prior to admission of the medication. (b) Assess maternal BP, respirations, pulse, and FHR status. (c) Laboring woman is able to rest between contractions and has increased comfort.

38. Transition phase of the first stage of labor.

39. (a) Nursing interventions may include the following: Stand close by with your face near to hers and talk to her very quietly in a supportive voice (e.g., "I will stay with you, breathe with me, watch me, take a breath, your contraction is ending, take a cleansing breath and rest"); do not touch her (in transition women do not usually like to be touched); keep the environment quiet to decrease stimulation; provide support and encouragement to both partners; demonstrate confidence in your abilities to assist the couple; do not leave her alone; be accepting and nonjudgmental of her coping skills, but do not

allow her to hurt another person (e.g., biting her support person). All of these nursing interventions are aimed at increasing support, comfort, trust, and rapport, and providing a caring and supportive environment. (b) The woman is able to rest between contractions, is exhibiting less panicky behavior, is able to breathe with contractions, appears to have increased comfort, is less restless, has relaxed her face and body.

40. (a) Hyperventilation (breathing too fast and deeply with contractions). (b) Talk with her and encourage her to slow her respirations; breathe with her; have her cup her hands in around her mouth and breathe in and out in her hands during contractions, and breathe into a paper bag. You must remember that the woman is experiencing an acute sense that she must breathe faster and deeper, and it is difficult for her to believe that she needs to change that pattern. Stay with her and provide encouragement and support until the pattern improves. (c) See Table 20–6, p. 560.

41. (a) 10, (b) second stage

42. Signs include uncontrollable urge to bear down, increased bloody show, bulging of the perineum, crowning of the fetal head.

43. See text, pp. 565–567; and Table 20–9, p. 567

44. See text, p. 000

45. Provide continuous encouragement for resting between contractions, provide support during pushing efforts, keep couple informed of progress, provide comfort measures (cool cloth over forehead, ice chips, privacy, assistance with positioning and support of body parts).

46. Indications include a short perineum that appears that it will tear during birth, and the need to enlarge the vaginal opening for the use of forceps or a vacuum extractor to hasten the second stage.

47. See text, Figure 23–3, p. 666

48. See text, pp. 665–667

49. *Prenatal:* exercise, tailor sitting, massage the perineum with oil. *Labor and birth:* allow the mother to respond to the natural urge to push instead of encouraging her to push before she feels a strong urge (work with her body, not the desires of attending nurses and physician/ CNM). During pushing, stretch the perineum slightly by massaging gently with gloved fingers and warmed solution. Encourage the woman to respond to what her body is directing her to do and to push as much as she feels comfortable. Encourage gentle pushing when the fetal head is born.

50. To prevent the fetal head from emerging rapidly and tearing the vaginal tissues.

51. To remove secretions that have filled the fetal mouth, nose, and throat.

52. (a) Circle assessments in Figures 11–5. (b) The Apgar score is 8. One point off for respiratory effort and one point off for color. (c) Apgar scores are assessed at 1 and 5 minutes past birth.

53. A pink body indicates that the baby's heartbeat and respirations are in the normal range, and the baby is probably not having difficulty. You could probably assume that the heart rate would be scored 2, and the respiratory effort would also meet the criteria for a score of 2. As long as the baby has not received any narcotics or medications that cause muscle relaxation, you could also assume that the baby will have a 2 on muscle tone and reflex irritability.

Overall, the heart rate and then respirations are the most important factors because without them the other characteristics are not possible. Think about it: you cannot have a pink body and depressed or no respirations, and you certainly cannot have an absence of heartbeat.

54. Dry newborn with warmed blankets, place newborn skin to skin on mother's chest, place under radiant heater.

55. To prevent evaporative heat loss.

56. The radiant heater works by warming the surface that the heat touches; therefore, the newborn should be unclothed so the skin is warmed.

57. (a) The umbilical vessels and the kidneys are formed embryonically at about the same time. The absence of one artery may indicate kidney problems. (b) Two arteries and one vein should be present.

58. Answers include application of name bands, footprinting.

59. Head slightly down with head to the side.

60. Stimulation of the vagus nerve in the back of the throat with subsequent bradycardia.

61. The brief physical assessment of the newborn should include overall size and general appearance; posture and movements; rate and irregularities of the apical pulse; respirations (rate, presence of retractions, grunting).

    If the newborn is stable, you may continue by assessing the head (general appearance, discoloration, fontanelles, flaring of nostrils, condition of palate); the neck (webbing or any limitation of movement); the abdomen (size, shape, contour, abnormal pulsations, number of vessels in umbilical cord); extremities (asymmetry, movement, number of digits); skin (discolorations, edema); elimination (record on newborn record any voiding or stools).

62. Place newborn baby skin to skin on mother's chest, encourage the mother and father to touch their baby, provide support in interacting with the baby (the environment in the birthing/delivery room may suggest that the parents need to "not touch"), point out similarities of the baby to the parents.

63. Talking to the baby; stroking, patting, and holding the baby; talking in a higher voice; looking for similarities with family members; calling the baby by name; snuggling; *en face* position; looking for eye contact.

64. Further protrusion of the umbilical cord out of the vagina, a gush of vaginal bleeding, a change in the shape of the uterus, a rise of the fundus in the abdomen.

65. (a) Schultze expulsion results in the center of the placenta separating from the endometrial wall; the rest of the placenta is therefore pulled off. The Duncan separation begins with a margin of the center separating; then the rest of the placenta is pulled off. (b) A Schultze placenta appears with the fetal side (shiny). With a Duncan separation, the maternal side (more rough and ragged looking because it is the cotyledons) shows.

66. A Duncan placenta may leave small fragments of the cotyledons still attached to the endometrial wall. This leads to inadequate uterine contractions and postpartal bleeding.

67. Assessment of the placenta should include the following: (a) examination of membranes: a missing section may indicate retention of a piece of membrane in the uterus, and vessels traversing the membranes may indicate placenta succenturiate. (b) Inspection of the umbilical cord for number of vessels, insertion site, and abnormalities, such as knots. (c) Inspection of the placenta for missing cotyledons, infarcts, and/or areas of calcification, and overall size and weight.

68. (a) Pitocin promotes rhythmic uterine contractions and assists in preventing uterine bleeding in the early postpartum time. (b) Assess maternal BP. See Drug Guide: Oxytocin (Pitocin).

69. (a) First stage: 8 hours. (b) Second stage: 1 hour 10 minutes. (c) Third stage: 15 minutes. (d) Fourth stage: began at 5:25 PM and lasted until 7:25 or 9:25 PM (2–4 hours)

70. See text, Table 18–5, p. 486.

71. a

72. c

73. a

74. a

75. b

76. a

77. a

78. a

79. a

80. a

81. a

82. When the uterus is not firmly contracting, the muscles become soft and blood collects in the uterus. A boggy uterus needs to be gently massaged until it is firm.

83. Comfort measures include cold pack to perineum, positioning, and pain medications if needed.

84. At the end of the recovery period the vital signs should be stable; the uterine fundus is in the midline, is firm, and is at the level of the umbilicus or 1–2 fingerbreadths (1–2 fb) below; the perineum is not excessively swollen or bruised; the episiotomy is not excessively swollen or bruised; and the skin edges are well approximated. If the woman has had regional anesthesia, she has usually regained sensation in the affected parts. In some hospitals, the recovery period does not end until the new mother has voided.

85. (a) First stage: hypoxia of uterine muscle cells during contractions, stretching of the lower

uterine segment and cervix, dilatation of the cervix, and pressure on adjacent structures. (b) Second stage: hypoxia of contracting uterine muscle cells, distention of the vagina and perineum, and pressure on adjacent structures. (c) Third stage: uterine contractions and cervical dilatation as the placenta is expelled.

86.    See text, pp. 493–494

87.    (a) The woman is willing to receive medication; vital signs are stable. (b) The FHR is between 120 and 160 beats/minute, and no decelerations are present; the fetus exhibits normal movement; the fetus is at term; meconium staining is not present. (c) The contraction pattern is well established; the cervix is dilated at least 5–6 cm in nulliparas and 3–4 cm in multiparas; the fetal presenting part is engaged; there is progressive descent of the fetal presenting part. No complications are present.

88.    (a) Active phase; 7 cm; Barbara cries out and is restless, repeatedly changes positions, blood pressure and pulse increased, FHR 140. (b) It is difficult to identify the three top nursing considerations that all nurses would agree on. However, we suggest that the top three would be: (1) assess the woman's history and present status to identify contraindications for administering analgesics, (2) determine that the woman is not hypotensive and fetal status is normal (FHR is in normal range with average variability and no variable or late decelerations), and (3) ensure that the ordered medication is appropriate and the dosage is within the expected range. The next two nursing considerations would be as follows: provide client safety after administration (e.g., ensure that side rails on bed are up, assist with all movement from bed, place call bell within reach) and reassess the woman and her fetus approximately 15 minutes after IM injection and 5 minutes after IV administration to ensure normal effects and to identify quickly untoward effects. Were your top three within the top five that we selected?

89.    (a) In active labor, the physician may administer an epidural block. (b) In the second stage, the physician may administer a pudendal block or local anesthetic.

90.    d

91.    *Actions:* The immediate assessment should include looking at the perineum and performing a sterile vaginal examination if the head is not already visible.
       *Actions:* While placing your gloved hand on the perineum just under the vagina to provide support to the perineal tissues, ask Carolyn to push once more. As soon as the baby's head is born, ask Carolyn to pant. The panting will allow you a moment to suction the baby's mouth with a bulb syringe and to check quickly for a nuchal cord.
       *Actions:* You will slide your finger up along the side of the baby's head to feel for a loop of umbilical cord around the baby's neck. If you find a loop, bend your finger at the first digit (making a "hook") and gently slip the cord over the baby's head.

92.    (a) abortion, (b) estimated date of birth, (c) electronic fetal monitor, (d) deceleration, (e) episiotomy, (f) fetal heart rate, (g) head circumference, (h) last menstrual period, (i) Rhesus factor, (j) rupture of membranes, (k) vaginal birth after cesarean

# 12 Answer Key

1. Anxiety and fear may be associated with fear of outcome, fear of performance or questions regarding ability to tolerate labor, fear of being hurt, anxiety regarding past experiences in the woman's life, inadequate knowledge, and lack of support. Anxiety may affect the labor by adding to the discomfort of uterine contractions and general body distress, making support and encouragement more difficult to accept, and slowing the labor and birth process.

2. Signs and symptoms of anxiety may include fearful looks on the face, numerous questions or reticence to interact with nurses and others, shaking, trembling, inability to access coping skills.

3. There are two thoughts that immediately come to mind. First, the couple may be presenting expected behaviors for their cultural group, and in this case, it is important to validate that the woman can be engaged and is not afraid to answer. You could say, "I need to ask another question, and this time it is important for you (the woman) to answer it for me." You can watch the interaction that occurs and whether she answers you directly or seems to wait for some sign of permission from the male partner. Second, the behaviors may indicate an abusive relationship in which the male is in control and the woman is silent and submissive. In this case, your first reaction will probably be to wish that you were not having this thought. It is not unusual for nurses and other people to have a suspicion but to not want to know the answer. It is uncomfortable and very awkward because you do not know what to do next. If you are an advocate for your client, it is important to talk with the woman in private. In a matter-of-fact tone, ask the partner to step out of the room. Ask the woman if she is safe (See assessment information on pages 106–107). If she indicates that she is in an abusive relationship, offer her support by asking if you can help, suggesting resources in the community, and asking if she would like to speak with social services. Ask how you can help her the most during labor and birth. Explain that you could not agree to anything that you believe might compromise her.

4. Failure to progress is frequently associated with a hypotonic labor pattern. The contractions decrease in frequency, duration, and intensity, and the fetal descent slows or stops. The laboring woman experiences discomfort, disappointment, anxiety, and stress.

5. The most important aspect of treatment is to rule out cephalopelvic disproportion. Once ruled out, IV oxytocin augmentation is usually started.

6. Precipitous labor and birth is one that begins and ends within 3 hours.

7. Treatment of a woman who has experienced precipitous labor will be to induce any subsequent births.

8. June 15

9. June 29

10. Postterm pregnancy is frequently associated with decreased amounts of amniotic fluid, which sets the stage for compression of the umbilical cord. When compression of the cord is present, a variable deceleration of the FHR occurs. Other problems may include meconium aspiration and intrauterine growth retardation.

11. An amnioinfusion is a technique by which approximately 250–300 mL of warmed, sterile, saline or lactated Ringer's solution is introduced into the uterine cavity after membranes have ruptured (spontaneously or by amniotomy). The desired effect is to instill an adequate amount of fluid in order to relieve any pressure on the umbilical cord, which is indicated by the cessation of variable decelerations.

12. Other nursing interventions would be to change the woman's position.

13. During each variable deceleration, the fetus may be stressed and may release meconium into the amniotic fluid, which stains the fluid a light blackish-green. With continued fetal stress, a larger amount of meconium may be released, making the amniotic fluid thicker and more discolored. Aspiration of the meconium-stained fluid can cause meconium aspiration pneumonitis after birth.

14. Indications for induction of labor include previous precipitous labor, postterm pregnancy, preexisting maternal disease (diabetes, PIH), premature rupture of membranes (PROM), chorioamnionitis, fetal demise, IUGR, mild abruptio placentae.

15. A positive CST means that late decelerations are present with uterine contractions. In this case, inducing labor would compromise the fetus.

16. Additional contraindications include client refusal, placenta previa, abnormal fetal presentation, prolapsed cord, prior classic uterine incision, active genital herpes, and cephalopelvic disproportion (CPD).

17. The Bishop score describes characteristics of the cervix and fetal position and assigns a score to different findings. The higher the score, the more likely that labor is ready to occur. A score of 3 would not be conducive to successful induction at this time. A score of 9 or more is compatible with successful induction.

18. The correct answer is 6 mL/hour. To compute this problem you need to start with the following facts:

1 mL Pitocin = 10 units
1 unit = 1000 mU (milliunits)
10 units = 10,000 mU

$$\frac{10,000 \text{ mU}}{1000 \text{ mL}} = \frac{x}{1 \text{ mL}}$$

x = 10 mU/mL of intravenous fluid

There are 60 minutes in an hour, and you want 1 mU/minute; 60 min × 1 mU/min = 60 mU/hr. To obtain milliliters per hour:

$$\frac{10 \text{ mU}}{1 \text{ mL}} = \frac{60 \text{ mU}}{x \text{ mL}}$$

10x = 60
x = 6 mL/hr

Did you arrive at the correct answer? This problem requires a lot of thought, but it is important to be able to calculate Pitocin infusion rates so that the client's safety can be maintained.

19. Signs of water intoxication include nausea, vomiting, hypotension, tachycardia, cardiac arrhythmia.

20. Immediately prior to increasing the rate of intravenous Pitocin infusion, you must assess the following: maternal blood pressure and pulse, uterine contractions (frequency, duration, intensity), FHR (deviant patterns, variability), fetal response (excessive activity).

21. The problems that might occur in response to a Pitocin induction include tetanic contractions, late or variable decelerations in FHR, a significant increase or decrease in maternal blood pressure or pulse, signs of water intoxication if an electrolyte-free solution is used.

22. The sample fetal monitoring strip provides the following information: (a) The FHR baseline is 140 for the 8-minute segment. It is best to assess a 10-minute segment to accurately determine the baseline. (If you caught this point, congratulations. You had to know the definition of an FHR baseline and correctly count the spaces to realize that only 8 minutes are depicted.) (b) STV is present. (c) The variability is moderate. (d) Accelerations are not evident. (e) The contraction frequency is every 3 minutes. (f) The contraction duration is 60–75 seconds. (g) No. The infusion rate should not be advanced because "good" contractions have been achieved.

23. The strip indicates severe problems. (a) The immediate nursing actions would include discontinuing the Pitocin infusion and turning on the main intravenous line; turning the mother on her left side; starting oxygen administration at 6–10 L per minute; notifying the physician; anticipating preparations for effecting an immediate delivery. (b) The strip showed severe late decelerations with minimal variability and tetanic contractions every 1½ minutes lasting 80–90 seconds.

24. (a) Amniotomy is done to release amniotic fluid and allow the fetal presenting part (usually the occiput) to press more firmly on the cervix. This is thought to hasten labor. (b) First, the

FHR should be assessed immediately after the membranes have been ruptured. The rationale for this action is that the umbilical cord may wash down through the cervix as the amniotic fluid escapes. As pressure is exerted on the cord, the fetal blood supply may be compromised. Second, you need to assess the amniotic fluid for amount, color, and odor.

25. (a) Greenish color is probably meconium staining, although presence of a foul odor could indicate infection. (b) Reddish color indicates that blood is present in the amniotic fluid. (c) Foul odor is associated with an infection in the amniotic fluid.

26. The procedure is set up and administered in the same manner; however, response to the IV oxytocin is usually much quicker because uterine contractions are already occurring. The same assessments must be made.

27. Augmentation would be contraindicated in the following instances: in the presence of fetal distress; with strong suggestions of CPD; with hypertonic uterine contraction pattern; in the presence of placenta previa; with multiple gestation. It is questionable with vaginal birth following cesarean birth.

28. You will need to call the obstetrician and inform her or him of the contraindications you have found. Perhaps the physician was unaware of the presence of the contraindications. If the physician persists in ordering the augmentation, ask what it is about the contraindications that you are not clear on and how it will still be safe for the client. Perhaps there is information that you do not have. If the contraindications persist, you will need to clearly explain that it is outside of your agency policy and you will not be able to do it as it violates your agency standards and your standard of nursing practice. You will need to chart your conversation clearly in the client record and discuss this with your chain of command at this time.

29. d, e

30. f, g

31. a

32. b, c

33. (a) Frank breech, (b) complete breech, (c) single footling breech

34. The drawing should show the umbilical cord prolapsing down below the cervix.

35. (a) A prolapsed cord is susceptible to compression, which slows the blood flow to the fetus and results in a slowing of the fetal heart rate and variable decelerations. The fetus is not being perfused in an adequate manner and is at risk. (b) You would feel a pulsating cord. You must keep your examining fingers against the fetal presenting part and exert slight pressure upward to relieve pressure on the cord. Have the woman put on her call light; once assistance arrives, they can apply the fetal monitor to assess the effectiveness of your intervention. Usually a cesarean birth must occur rapidly to maximize the outcome for the fetus. (c) See Figure 12–5 on page 286.

36. (a) The following criteria should be present before an external version is done: a single fetus (multiple gestation fetuses may become entangled), the fetal breech is not engaged (engagement increases the difficulty of the version), intact amniotic membranes and adequate amount of fluid (diminished amounts of fluid make the fetus hard to move and may cause cord compression), fetal well-being should be evident as demonstrated by a reassuring FHR pattern and reactive NST. (b) See text, p. 000 (c) Some occult bleeding may occur during the version, and the woman could become sensitized at this time. (d) Pertinent areas to cover in discharge teaching include being aware of uterine contractions and the possible beginning of labor, leakage of clear fluid from the vagina (amniotic fluid), increased or decreased fetal movement (may be associated with fetal stress), vaginal bleeding (may be associated with placental bleeding), the reason for administering RhoGAM if it was given, the name and phone number of her physician in case there are further questions.

37. Signs and symptoms of twins include visualization of more than one gestational sac during ultrasound exam early in pregnancy, fundal height that exceeds the expected growth rate, and auscultation of two fetal heartbeats at least 10 bpm apart in rate.

38. Antepartal problems may include physical discomfort, dyspnea on exertion, PIH, urinary

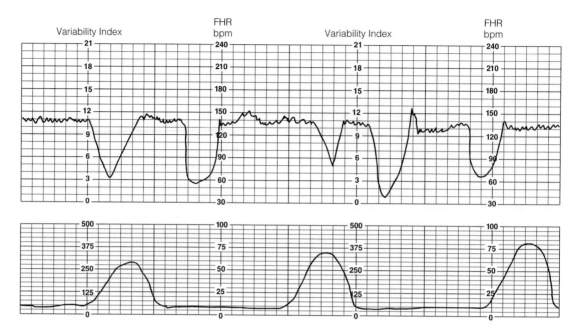

**Figure 12–5**

tract infections, backaches, preterm labor, placenta previa, abruptio placentae, prolapsed cord and hemorrhage during birth and postpartum.

39. Treatment plan will include areas such as increased nutritional intake, increased rest, increased antepartal monitoring (visits, antepartal testing).

40. Implications for the fetuses may include inadequate nourishment of one fetus during gestation; premature labor, with associated problems of respiratory distress syndrome; difficulty in evaluating whether the second fetus can be delivered vaginally if the first fetus is delivered breech; interlocked fetuses; slow or interrupted labor because of overstretching of the uterus.

41. If one fetus exhibits problems, treatment must be initiated quickly in the same manner as it would if only one fetus were present.

42. Fetal distress would be indicated by any of the following: loss of variability, severe late or variable decelerations, severe bradycardia, meconium staining in a vertex presentation, cessation of movement, hyperactive fetal movement.

43. (a) postpartal bleeding and hemorrhage, (b) this occurs because of overstretching of the uterus

and inadequate uterine contractions following birth.

44. You should suspect a breech presentation.

45. When the fetus is in a breech presentation, there may be a release of meconium due to the pressures occurring during contractions. In this instance, the release of meconium would most likely be viewed as physiologic. However, the possibility of fetal distress must be considered.

When there is evidence of meconium staining of the amniotic fluid during labor, the birth team needs to be prepared to remove secretions from the newborn's naso-oropharynx immediately after birth. Suction is frequently used to remove these secretions. In the case of a breech presentation, the newborn will be suctioned as soon as the head is delivered. In vertex presentation, the naso-oropharynx is suctioned as soon as the head appears, and before the first breath is taken, so that the secretions are not drawn into the lungs with the first breath. The vocal cords will be visualized with a laryngoscope. If meconium is seen, suctioning will be done. Aspiration of meconium can result in meconium aspiration pneumonia in the early neonatal period.

46. (a) This is a very difficult situation. Anna deserves straight, honest information. You might say something like, "I'm very sorry, Anna. I did not hear your baby's heartbeat. Your doctor is on the way. May I sit with you while we wait?"

As a student, you may have fears that you will not hear the FHR and mistakenly think the baby is dead. In reality, you will be assessing FHR with your instructor or with birthing room staff. When you are just learning to listen to FHR and you either are not able to hear the FHR at all or are not sure what you are hearing, you might say to the nurse, "I'm not as experienced as you in listening to the FHR, and I'm not sure what I'm hearing. Would you listen to it now, please?" (b) In this situation, it is not unusual to feel very scared and anxious. Part of your mind is telling you that the baby may be dead and another part is saying "no" it can't be true, and if it is true, it can't be happening now, to you. The first feelings are most like anxiety and dread. All these feelings are common in this situation. It is important to recognize your feelings and know that they are normal and to be expected.

47. See text, pp. 633–634

48. Abruptio placentae is separation of the placenta before birth of the fetus. The types are marginal, central, and complete.

49. Placenta previa is implantation of the placenta in the lower uterine segment or down over the internal cervical os. The placenta precedes the fetus. The types are low-lying, marginal, and complete.

50. b, d, f

51. c, e, f

52. a, d

53. See text, pp. 634–637

54. No vaginal exam. In doing an exam, you may puncture one of the cotyledons and precipitate bleeding.

55. Dyspnea, cyanosis, cardiovascular collapse, shock, coma, and death. (a) A difficult, rapid labor. (b) See text, pp. 645–646

56. 2000

57. Backache from increased weight in uterus and back strain; difficulty breathing from increased pressure upward on the diaphragm; increased edema in feet, ankles, and legs due to increased pressure on vessels on lower extremities. See text for self-care measures.

58. Esophageal atresia that diminishes or prevents fetal swallowing may be identified by ultrasound. Kidney disorders that affect the fetal kidney output may be identified by ultrasound. Maternal diabetes, which affects the fetal urine output, is identified by maternal testing.

59. The uterus decompressed in size rapidly with the loss of a great amount of amniotic fluid. This may precipitate a change in the size of the uterus and the placenta may separate.

60. Oligohydramnios is defined as a severely decreased amount of concentrated amniotic fluid.

61. Variable decelerations, due to inadequate fluid that allows the umbilical cord to float without compression.

62. There is a decreased amount of fluid swallowed and urine produced and excreted by the fetus.

63. The maternal pelvis is greatly diminished in size. She will most likely need to have a cesarean birth.

64. Pelvic measurements would be obtained during antenatal care; while in labor, a clinical pelvimetry or x-ray pelvimetry may be done.

65. A TOL may be attempted in an effort to avoid an unnecessary cesarean birth. The woman would be induced or would come in when labor occurs and her progress would be closely watched in terms of uterine contractions, fetal status, and especially fetal descent.

66. Cervical dilatation in a primigravida is approximately 1.2 cm/hr; 1.5 cm/hr in a multigravida.

67. Fetal descent should be progressive from –3 to 0 and then +1 to +4 for vaginal birth.

68. Failure of cervix to dilate, failure of fetal descent, maternal pushing for greater than 2 hr (primigravida) or 3 hr (multigravida).

69. A gestation with a very large baby or a malposition (such as brow) that is larger than the maternal pelvis will accommodate. If the subsequent fetus is smaller, a vaginal birth may be possible.

70. Indications include maternal heart disease, maternal exhaustion, fetal stress or distress.

71. Complete dilatation of the cervix, known fetal station and position, ruptured membranes.

72. See text, p. 668

73. Maternal risks include lacerations of the birth canal and perineum, increased bleeding. Fetal/neonatal risks include caput succedaneum or cephalhematoma, facial bruising, swelling or abrasions, transient facial paralysis.

74. Nursing interventions that are necessary during a forceps-assisted birth include the following: Explain the procedure to the woman and her support person. Encourage the woman to maintain her breathing pattern during application of the forceps. (Panting may help to relieve the "need to push" sensation that she will feel as the forceps are applied.) Monitor the FHR continuously. Monitor contractions. Inform the physician when a contraction begins and ends, because he or she will exert downward pressure on the forceps during a contraction. Provide support to the woman throughout the process. Ensure that adequate resuscitation equipment is available and in working order before the birth. After birth, assess the newborn for Apgar score; facial bruising, swelling, abrasions, and/or paralysis; signs of cerebral trauma; and movement of arms (to detect paralysis).

75. The bruising and swelling will slowly go away, and there will not be any lasting effects for their baby.

76. (a) The vacuum extractor is devised to apply negative pressure on the fetal occiput so that traction may be applied to the extractor, and the fetus is assisted in the birth. (b) The negative pressure that builds up in the cup draws the fetal scalp up and edema forms in the tissues. The "chignon" is an area of swelling (caput) that is the size and shape of the extractor cup. (c) The parents need to know the reason the extractor is needed and the expected effects, benefits, and risks for both the mother and fetus/neonate. The mother's permission needs to be verbally obtained.

77. (a) Shave the maternal abdomen from the umbilicus downward to just over the symphysis. (b) The indwelling bladder catheter is inserted in the same manner as for other adults, with the exception that identification of the urethral meatus may be more difficult because of swelling of the vulvar tissues and that actual insertion of the catheter may take more pressure because the fetal head is down against the vulvar tissues. (c) See text, pp. 673–676

78. 37.5

79. See text, p. 674

80. See text, pp. 674–675

81. If your teaching has been effective, Janel will understand the need to move her legs frequently during the recovery phase, she will take deep breaths and cough while splinting her abdomen with a pillow, she will ask for pain medication when she feels she needs it, she will cooperate with the turning and changing of position every 2 hours, and she will cooperate with ambulation to facilitate return of bowel motility.

82. As your mind races, searching for the "correct" response, remember that there are many ways to answer. Although you may be tempted to offer her reassurances that she is not a failure, this is a nontherapeutic approach. It will be helpful to focus on the "feeling" components that Janel seems to be expressing. Possible responses may be: "When the birth doesn't occur as you have planned, sometimes it feels like something is missing," or "When things don't happen as you plan, it feels as if something is wrong," or "It's hard to feel as if you've failed."

Each of these possible responses focuses in on the feelings she may be expressing. It lets her know you have heard her and are willing to talk.

83. The father's comfort can be enhanced by answering any questions that he has, providing information regarding the cesarean birth, and describing ways in which he may want to be involved. See further discussion in text, pp. 675–676.

84. (a) Contraindications would include a previous classic uterine incision, inability to perform a cesarean within 30 minutes, client refusal. (b) Becky needs to present with a history of not more than two previous cesareans. The previous uterine incisions should not be classic incisions. During labor, the maternal assessment would include vital signs for early detection of

hemorrhage, uterine contraction pattern for normal contraction characteristics, and fetus for reassuring FHR pattern.

85. Of the three choices, "insufficient data" was the correct choice. The abdominal incision and the uterine incision do not necessarily match. The only way to validate the type of uterine incision is to review the surgical record of the first cesarean birth. If the uterine incision is a "classic" incision, a VBAC is usually contraindicated. If the type of uterine incision cannot be determined, many obstetricians would recommend a cesarean for any succeeding pregnancies.

86. (a) artificial rupture of membranes; (b) biparietal diameter; (c) cephalopelvic disproportion; (d) cesarean section; (e) elective low forceps; (f) disseminated intravascular coagulation; (g) hemolysis, elevated liver enzymes, low platelets; (h) intrauterine fetal death; (i) meconium staining of amniotic fluid; (j) Pitocin; (k) trial of labor; (l) vaginal birth after cesarean

# 13 Answer Key

1. (a) Mechanical: The baby's passage through the birth canal fosters removal of fluid from the lungs and throat. The chest recoil results in the taking in of air. When air is expelled against a partially closed glottis, it fosters an increase in pressure within the chest and opens alveoli. (b) Chemical stimuli: increase in $P_{CO_2}$ and decrease in oxygen triggers respiratory center. Prolonged asphyxia acts as a depressant. (c) Thermal stimuli: decrease in environment temperature stimulates skin nerve endings and rhythmic breathing. (d) Sensory stimuli: tactile (thorough drying), auditory, and visual.

2. The newborn's cardiovascular system accomplishes the following anatomic and physiologic alterations during the transition from fetal to neonatal circulation: increase in aortic pressure and decrease in venous pressure as a result of loss of the placenta; increased systemic pressure and decreased pulmonary artery pressure due to decreased pulmonary circulatory resistance and vasodilation; closure of the ductus venosus and foramen ovale; closure of the ductus arteriosis, which increases blood flow in the pulmonary vascular system.

3. a

4. Flexed position, to decrease exposed surface area and decrease heat losses.

5. Physiologic jaundice usually appears about the second or third day of life. Jaundice is the yellow color that can be seen in the newborn's eyes and skin. It comes from normal breakdown of RBCs and the liver's decreased ability to process and excrete bilirubin, which results in a temporary buildup of bilirubin in the blood and fatty tissue under the skin. It is usually gone by the 10th to 14th day of life. The time of onset is important to note because it will help you differentiate jaundice that is considered pathologic when it occurs at birth or within the first 24 hours after birth.

6. See text, pp. 702–703

7. a

8. a

9. (a) 38, (b) 39

10. See text, p. 715, Figure 25–1

11. Factors that can influence a neonate's gestational age score are: (a) Medications (especially on the assessment of the neurologic components). (b) Anoxia or hypoxia, which can result in decreased muscle tone and reflex determinations. (c) Timing of the scoring. For example, if sole creases are evaluated after 12 hours, the natural drying of the soles increases what appear to be sole creases; or if the birthing room nurse thoroughly removes the vernix before the gestational score is determined, the score will be inaccurate. (d) Variations in the usual physical characteristics because of intrauterine conditions. For example, the infant of a diabetic mother and the premature large-for-gestational-age infant both have more breast tissue (increased subcutaneous tissue) than an infant of true gestational maturation. (e) Difficult birth, which may make determination of skull firmness difficult.

12. To anticipate possible physiologic problems and establish an individualized plan of newborns and their families.

13. (a) 97.5–99.0F (36.4–37.2C) axillary; (b) 120–160 bpm (100 asleep, 180 crying); (c) 30–60 breaths/min; (d) 80–60/45–40 mmHg; (e) 3405 g (7 lb, 8 oz Caucasian, varies with ethnicity); (f) 50 cm (20 in), range 48–52 cm (18–22 in); (g) 32–37 cm (12.5–14.5 in); (h) 32 cm (12.5 in), range 30–35cm (12–14 in)

14. See text, p. 717, Figure 25–14

15. 5–10

16. Small fluid intake, increased volume of meconium stooling, fluid shifts, and increased urination.

17. Place infant flat on the back with legs extended as much as possible; if breech delivery, remeasure

when legs are no longer in the in utero breech position.

18. See text, pp. 719–721
19. b
20. See text, pp. 726–727
21. See text, p. 734–748
22. See text, p. 733, Table 25–5
23. Answers may include the following reflexes: yawn, blink, cough/ sneeze, gag, withdrawal from painful stimuli.
24. See text, pp. 734–748
25. Decreased peripheral circulation, which results in vasomotor instability and capillary stasis, can be seen as acrocyanosis.
26. As the newborn nurse, you should ascertain the following essential areas of information from the birthing room nurse: previously identified perinatal risk factors; problems occurring during labor and birth, such as signs of fetal distress or maternal problems (abruptio placentae, preeclampsia, and prolapse of the cord, all of which compromise the fetus in utero); medications given to the mother during labor or given to the newborn in the immediate postbirth period; the baby's Apgar scores; resuscitative measures administered to the newborn; elimination during the postbirth period (did the newborn void or pass meconium in the birthing room?); general condition and activity level. If you identified these areas, you have a basis for identifying significant potential problems for the newborn. These areas of information provide a database from which to make continued careful and significant observations and nursing diagnoses during the transitional period.
27. Nursing actions that you would perform initially and during the first 4 hours after birth would be as follows: assessing for any signs of neonatal distress; noting vital signs (including blood pressure in some agencies); measuring weight; measuring length; taking head and chest circumference measurements; administering prophylactic medications; scoring for gestational age; do blood work (Hct and heelstick glucose) at 4 hours of age. In addition, many institutions do a general head-to-toe admission physical. Other institutions may also do stomach aspirations, but this

procedure is controversial and shouldn't be done until the newborn is stable because it can cause bradycardia and apnea.

28. Absence of normal intestinal bacterial flora needed to synthesis vitamin K results in low levels of vitamin K. This creates a transient blood coagulation deficiency between the second and fifth day of life.
29. *Actions:* Immediately after Glen's birth, you would dry him off, assess the heart and respiratory rates, determine the 1 and 5 minute Apgar scores, and then do a quick physical assessment for congenital anomalies.
   *Actions:* Place Glen skin-to-skin with his mother. Cover them both with a warm blanket to assist in maintaining his temperature. Assist Glen to suckle at the breast, and provide any support Glen and his mom may need to facilitate the bonding process.
30. 0.5–1 mg IM in the middle one-third of the vastus lateralis.
31. (a) Ophthalmic neonatorum, (b) *Neisseria gonorrhoeae*
32. Answers may include: 1-percent silver nitrate, 0.5-percent erythromycin, or 1-percent tetracycline
33. Per agency format
34. Polycythemia, increase fluid intake; anemia, observe for any respiratory distress; jaundice, assess need for phototherapy; hypoglycemia, observe for signs of jitteriness and temperature instability and initiate early feedings (breast milk or glucose water).
35. A possible nursing diagnosis would be *Ineffective Airway Clearance.* You would immediately aspirate the mouth and nasal pharynx with a bulb syringe, holding the newborn with its head down and neck extended to facilitate drainage as you aspirate the mucus. If you also recognize an increase in mucus production during the second period of reactivity, you are becoming alert and prepared to intervene in this very real problem.
36. Daily neonatal assessments should include (a) vital signs, (b) weight, (c) overall color, (d) stool pattern, (e) voiding pattern, (f) caloric and fluid intake, (g) cord care.

37. Per agency format
38. Urine is straw colored and odorless; may be cloudy with mucus strands; will have increased specific gravity and decreased output until oral intake increases.
39. Check chart and see whether Ryan voided at birth. Assess for adequacy of fluid intake, bladder distention, restlessness, and signs of discomfort. Notify appropriate clinical personnel.
40. Within 12–24 hours or at least by 48 hours of life. First stools are meconium, which are thick, tarlike, and dark green-black.
41. The nursing diagnosis: **Knowledge Deficit** related to lack of information about breastfeeding correctly might apply. Ms Montoya is obviously eager to be successful but has many unanswered questions. Her statement, even though not phrased as a request, was her way of reaching out and asking for assistance.
42. See text, pp. 785–790
43. See text, pp. 790–794, Table 24-4 pp. 795–796
44. Because women are often discharged within 24 hours of delivery, it is difficult to effectively complete infant care teaching. You can help reinforce Ms Montoya's learning by presenting material in different ways (verbal instruction followed by practice, for example, or by showing a videotape followed by discussion). You can then reinforce positive behaviors. For example, if you observe Ms Montoya using the football hold, you might say, "I think it's really wise of you to try using the different feeding positions. Can you feel the difference in the suction when your baby is in this position?" When she is ready to leave, it is always helpful to provide handouts with specific information so the new mother will have a practical reference at home. By the same token, Ms Montoya may find it helpful to have the phone number of the mother-baby unit so she can call someone if questions arise.
45. Your teaching plan will have been effective if Ms Montoya is able to successfully breastfeed her infant and demonstrate the techniques you have covered. For the cognitive content covered, you can ask Ms Montoya to describe to you the information you have shared. You can then discuss it briefly to learn whether she understands it fully.
46. The adequacy of the fluid and caloric intake of a breastfed infant is determined by weighing him or her before and after nursing and by observing the quantity of urine and feces and their patterns of elimination.
47. It is not uncommon for newborns to have decreased intake and weight loss in the first week of life. By the end of the first week, the newborn should regain weight and start gaining weight at about 1 oz/day for the first 6 months. Intake should not exceed 32 oz/day. Ascertain how much Christy is eating and encourage her mother to offer the bottle at least every 3–4 hours.
48. See text, pp. 799–800
49. c
50. Based on information in Chapters 25–26 in the textbook, formulate an informative and supportive response to these mothers' questions and concerns.
51. Ascertain whether the parents have any questions and whether they have signed the permit based on information; gather equipment and prepare newborn by removing diaper; provide for topical anesthetic before procedure and pain medication after as needed; provide comfort measures during and after procedure; apply Vaseline with diaper changes; assess for adequacy of voiding; and assess for bleeding.
52. d
53. Cleanse the penis daily, but do not attempt to retract the foreskin.
54. Essential components of a newborn discharge teaching program would include the following: bathing (skin, scalp, and nail care), eye and ear care, nasal suctioning (use of a bulb syringe), cord care, circumcision care or care of the uncircumcised male infant, care of female genitalia, diapering, positioning and handling, etablishing a feeding schedule versus feeding on demand, burping, pumping the breasts and supplemental feeding for breastfed infants, formula preparation, introduction to solids (what, when, why), providing vitamin supplements, stooling

and voiding patterns, sleep patterns, self-soothing methods, clothing, neonatal behavioral changes that may occur after discharge, observation for signs of illness, use of the thermometer, testing for phenylketonuria, pediatric follow-up.

55. a

56. a

57. d

58. See text pp. 772–773

59. a

60. See text p. 768, Table 26–3

61. (a) abdominal circumference, (b) brown adipose tissue, (c) chest circumference, (d) head circumference, (e) phenylketonuria

# 14    Answer Key

1.  Answers may include exposure to environmental hazards; low socioeconomic level; preexisting maternal condition such as diabetes, age, or parity; gestational diseases; pregnancy complications.

2.  Baby Joey's gestational age is 36–37 weeks, which places him as being preterm, and his weight of 1500 g places him below the tenth percentile for weight. His GA and weight classify him as a preterm SGA newborn. Based on this classification, you would want to watch Joey for the potential problems of hypothermia, respiratory distress, hypoglycemia, hypocalcemia, and polycythemia.

3.  postterm

4.  preterm

5.  large for gestational age

6.  small for gestational age

7.  d

8.  Answers may include primiparity or grand-multiparity, small stature, PIH, substance abuse, lack of prenatal care, smoking, age <16 or >40 yrs.

9.  Any infant who at birth is at or below the tenth percentile on intrauterine growth charts should be suspected of being small for gestational age. If growth retardation is the result of an acute episode of placental insufficiency, observe the infant for loss of subcutaneous fat and muscle mass; a wide-eyed face; loss of vernix prior to full term; dry and desquamated skin; and the presence of a meconium-stained cord, skin, and nails in a full-term or preterm infant. By your identification of a possible SGA infant, you can be instrumental in meeting his or her immediate special needs and in reducing the possible long-term sequelae.

10. Perinatal asphyxia, aspiration syndrome, hypothermia, hypoglycemia, hypocalcemia, and polycythemia.

11. IDM babies are LGA, macrosomic, and may be plethoric: they have large placentas and umbilical cords.

12. Caused by exposure to high levels of maternal glucose and an increase in fetal secretion of insulin.

13. Serum glucose levels on cord blood, hourly for first 4 hours, then every 4 hours until stable.

14. 1–3 hours

15. 40

16. Some signs and symptoms of hypoglycemia include lethargy or jitteriness, poor feeding, vomiting, temperature instability, apnea or irregular respirations.

17. Early detection and ongoing monitoring of signs of hypoglycemia and polycythemia; provision of adequate caloric intake with breast milk or formula and infusion of glucose as ordered.

18. d

19. c

20. Answers may include birth trauma, hyperbilirubinemia, hypocalcemia, congenital birth defects.

21. Obstetric situations that would lead you to suspect a postterm pregnancy include the following: oligohydramnios, weight loss of 3 lb or more per week in the last weeks of pregnancy, meconium-stained amniotic fluid in a full-term infant, palpation of a hard fetal head, high fetal head arrest, and prolonged labor due to uterine inertia or CPD. Women of high parity (gravida 4 or more), primigravidas, and women whose preceding pregnancy was postterm are also more prone to go beyond term in their present pregnancy.

22. Dry, cracked, parchment-like skin without vernix, long fingernails, profuse scalp hair, long thin body, alert appearance possibly from chronic intrauterine hypoxia, yellow-stained skin and cord.

23. d
24. Answers may include hypoglycemia, meconium aspiration, polycythemia, seizures, hypothermia.
25. Answers may include maternal disease such as cardiac, renal, diabetes, PIH, cervical incompetence, infections; substance abuse, multiple fetuses, fetal infections, hydramnios; low socioeconomic level, poor prenatal care; history of preterm births.
26. b
27. The three initial assessments you should make on the arrival of a preterm newborn in the nursery area are as follows: observation of signs of respiratory distress, core temperature determination to assess whether hypothermia or cold stress will complicate this infant's course, and gestational age determination to identify other potential problems. You may have identified other areas, but these are the essential ones. Refer to your textbook if you had any difficulty identifying the initial needs of the preterm newborn.
28. b
29. a
30. d
31. See text, pp. 828–829
32. See text, pp. 823–824, and Procedure 28–1
33. (a) Nursing assessments of Mariah's tolerance of gavage feedings would include observing for any degree of abdominal distention during or after the feeding; a formula residual of less than 1 mL prior to the next feeding; lack of regurgitation; and no apnea, bradycardia, cyanosis, or color changes. A program of alternate gavage and nipple feeding is recommended to decrease the possibility of fatigue during feeding. (b) Active sucking motions during and between feedings might indicate the preterm infant's readiness for nipple feeding. You would expect the preterm infant who could tolerate nipple feedings to have a weak grasp of the nipple but a strong suck and to show satiety and relief of oral tension as she feeds.
34. d
35. See text, pp. 830–831
36. See text, pp. 830, 853–858
37. See text, pp. 831–832, 858–859
38. Some complications associated with cocaine-exposed infants include poor state organization and decreased interactive behaviors, congenital malformations, withdrawal, motor development problems.
39. See text, pp. 835–836, Table 28–2
40. b
41. c
42. Needs may include comfort measures such as swaddling and small frequent feedings.
43. c
44. See text, p. 841
45. b
46. (a) acquired immunodeficiency syndrome, (b) fetal alcohol effects, (c) fetal alcohol syndrome, (d) infant of diabetic mother, (e) infant of substance abusing mother, (f) intrauterine growth retardation, (g) large for gestational age, (h) small for gestational age

# 15 Answer Key

1. b
2. (a) Meconium aspiration syndrome (MAS); (b) oropharynx, then nasopharynx are suctioned via low-pressure wall suction; (c) if thick meconium is present, clinician may visualize glottis and suction meconium from trachea.
3. If you answered "no," you were correct. Celeste is not a candidate for further resuscitation because of her vigorous crying after birth, no signs of respiratory distress, and the thin nature of the meconium-stained amniotic fluid. Vigorous resuscitation with intubation is controversial in this situation as it may do more harm to the baby.

   Your most pressing nursing goal is to dry off the baby and continue assessment of respiratory function.
4. Vigorous suctioning can stimulate the vagus nerve and cause bradycardia.
5. (a) 15–25, (b) 40–60
6. Brian probably has narcotic depression; you would give Narcan and continue ventilatory support.
7. b
8. d
9. Six signs of respiratory distress are tachypnea, inspiratory retractions, expiratory grunting, nasal flaring, cyanosis, and periods of apnea. Other signs you might look for after these six are lung rales or rhonchi, edema, and chin tug.
10. Congratulations if you scored Tricia's respiratory distress as 6. This is based on nasal flaring = 1, lower chest retractions = 1, xiphoid retractions = 1, chest lag on inspiration = 1, and expiratory grunting = 2.
11. A lower score is desirable for this scoring system and indicates normal respiratory effort or less respiratory distress. Tricia is having significant respiratory distress. Based on her small size and early gestational age, she is using large amounts of energy in her work of breathing and will exhaust her supply of surfactant.
12. Tricia's history of preterm delivery, a low Apgar score (hypoxic insult), and a low core temperature (cold stress) are all contributing factors to her development of respiratory distress syndrome.
13. To prevent drying of the mucous membranes and decrease action of the respiratory tract cilia.
14. Nursing responsibilities during oxygen administration include ensuring that the infant's head is under the oxygen hood and that respiratory passages are not obstructed, ensuring that the tubing is connected and free of moisture build-up, seeing that ambient oxygen concentrations are being monitored by oxygen sensors, and ensuring that oxygen delivery devices are calibrated periodically.
15. See text, p. 873, Table 29–2
16. c
17. The metabolic effects of cold stress include competition for albumin binding sites by increased nonesterified fatty acids, causing increased free circulating bilirubin; increased incidence of hypoglycemia resulting from glucose being used for thermogenesis; pulmonary vasoconstriction in response to the release of norepinephrine; and increase in oxygen consumption and metabolic acidosis as the body burns brown fat deposits. If you were successful in identifying these changes, you will also be aware that these changes may create serious life-threatening problems for an at-risk infant.
18. Warm baby slowly, monitor skin temperature, and maintain baby in a neutral thermal environment.
19. b
20. The three most prominent factors that influence the rate and amount of bilirubin conjugation are the following: rate of red blood cell

hemolysis, degree of liver maturity, and number of available albumin binding sites. In addition, you might remember that even after the bilirubin is conjugated, it can be unconjugated via the "enterohepatic circulation" and thus cause a delay in clearing the bilirubin from the circulatory system. Also, fetal red blood cells have a shorter half-life than adult red blood cells, which increases the rate of hemolysis.

21. Situations that alter the newborn's ability to conjugate bilirubin include the following: bacterial and viral infections; competition for albumin binding sites by drugs, particularly sulfa drugs and salicylates and nonesterified fatty acids; neonatal asphyxia, which decreases the binding affinity of biliribin to albumin; and the many causes of increased red blood cell hemolysis, such as cephalhematoma.

22. Some of the causes are fetal-neonatal asphyxia, hypothermia, hypoglycemia, maternal use of sulfa, aspirin, intracranial hemorrhage, and Rh-negative hemolytic disease; total bilirubin >15 mg/dL for preterm and >12.5 mg/dL for term newborns; occurs within the first 24 hours.

23. Your assessment of developing jaundice may be affected by fluorescent nursery lights with pink tints, which mask jaundice; by blue walls and blue blankets; and by the basic pigmentation of the gumline in ethnic people of color.

24. c

25. d

26. b

27. *Analysis:* You remember that one of the criteria for differentiating physiologic jaundice from pathologic jaundice is the time of onset. Because Alice is less than 24 hours old, it leads you to think the jaundice is pathologic in nature. Breastfeeding jaundice usually does not start until after three days. Sepsis is a possibility and requires further investigation.
*Actions:* Your nursing actions would include checking Alice's chart and her mother's chart for risk factors. As you check these charts, you find that her mother received no prenatal care, and the blood typing was done on admission. Alice's perinatal history reveals that the birth was normal without trauma, asphyxiation, or delay of the cord clamping. Alice was scored as a term AGA newborn. You complete your physical assessment to determine the extent of the jaundice and any other significant clinical findings such as activity state and bruising.
*Actions:* Laboratory data that you would expect to be evaluated include indirect and direct bilirubin, blood typing, Coombs' test on Alice's blood, complete white count, and RBC smear.

28. b

29. Some causes are prematurity, passage through the birth canal, premature rupture of maternal membranes, immature immune system of newborn, and invasive procedures.

30. Answers may include gram-negative organisms (*E. coli, Enterobacter, Proteus, Klebsiella*), gram-positive β-hemolytic streptococcus, coagulase-negative staphylococci.

31. a

32. Diagnostic tests that might be done as part of a septic work-up are primarily blood, spinal, nasopharyngeal, and urine cultures. If any lesions or reddened areas are noted, cultures from these areas should also be obtained. A complete blood count, chest x-ray, serology, and Gram stains of cerebrospinal fluid, urine, and umbilicus may also be required. Depending on the suspected cause of the sepsis, other tests may include x-rays of various portions of the body, serum IgM level determinations, and stomach (gastric) aspirations.

33. See text, pp. 898–899

34. a

35. (a) bronchopulmonary dysplasia, (b) meconium aspiration syndrome, (c) respiratory distress syndrome, (d) thermal neutral zone, (e) umbilical arterial catheterization

# 16 Answer Key

1. Postpartum is a time of major physiologic and psychologic adaptations as the body completes its adjustments following birth. The postpartal period lasts for 6 weeks.

2. Stage 4 (after the birth of the placenta to 1–4 hours past birth).

3. Cuddling and holding the baby, talking to the baby, stroking movements, smiling, *en face* position, seeking out eye contact, making soothing noises, asking questions about the baby are some examples.

4. Continue to provide opportunities for the parents to hold and interact with the baby. Complete any nursing activities while the baby is being held if at all possible, turn off the overhead lights to allow the baby to open his or her eyes, encourage the parents in their activities.

5. b

6. d

7. b

8. a

9. c

10. (a) Postpartal chill is usually experienced immediately after birth. It is thought to be related to the emptying of the uterus, the rapid cardiovascular changes that are occurring, and emotional responses to birth. (b) Postpartal diaphoresis occurs on the day of birth or the first postpartum day. The body needs to shed extra fluid that has been retained during the pregnancy. The new mother may wake up in the night drenched with perspiration. (c) *Afterpains* is a term used to refer to the rhythmic uterine contractions that continue to occur after birth. The contractions are essential for involution to occur.

11. It is a time of enormous readjustment and readaptation to role, family, and self-image.

12. The term *postpartum blues* refers to a feeling of depression and weepiness that many mothers experience in the first few days after birth.

13. See text, p. 912

14. The following essential areas need to be included in your daily physical assessment of the postpartal client: vital signs; breasts, including nipples; fundus and abdomen; lochia; perineum (including the anus); elimination; lower extremities; nutritional status; activity level.

    If you listed most of these, you are well on your way to providing good nursing care for your clients. If you missed three or more, you need to refer back to the postpartum section in your textbook. Other areas that may be considered are discomfort level and sleep patterns.

15. Note softness or firmness, filling, and engorgement. If woman is breastfeeding, note nipple soreness, cracking of nipples, and areas of firmness. This is also a good time to determine whether the mother does self-breast examinations and to provide teaching if she does not know how and desires to.

16. (a) To evaluate involution. (b) A full bladder may push the uterine fundus upward and to the maternal right side. The assessment will be inaccurate and palpating a full bladder will add to the mother's discomfort. (c) Place the palm of your hand at the level of the umbilicus and cup it back toward the maternal spine. Feel for a rounded, firm object. (d) Usually recorded as the number of fingerbreadths above or below the umbilicus.

17. Up toward the umbilicus and in the midline.

18. Lochia rubra, moderate amount, without clots.

19. Per agency policy

20. As she lies on her back, lochia collects in the vagina. When she stands, the collected lochia is discharged. As long as the uterus is firm and in the midline and the flow is not more than moderate, she is fine.

21. lateral Sims'

22. Observe for hemorrhoids

23. Bladder distention, amount of urine being voided, any difficulty or pain with voiding.

24. Whether she has had a bowel movement or not. What her normal bowel pattern is.

25. Teaching could include dietary needs for maintaining stool patterns and the need for rest, exercise, and adequate fluids. You can assess what the mother finds helpful to stimulate bowel movements.

26. To assess for bruising, edema, tenderness, redness, muscle strain, and thrombophlebitis.

27. By dorsiflexing the foot

28. *Analysis:* You suspect that Ms Jessup's bladder is distended. You know that because the uterine ligaments are still stretched, a distended bladder can easily displace the uterus and cause it to appear higher in the abdomen. It may also keep the uterus from remaining firmly contracted.
*Actions:* You assist Ms Jessup to the bathroom so she can attempt to void. You place a "Johnny cap" under the seat of the commode so you can measure her output. You show her where the call light is, and you leave her in privacy to attempt to void.
*Analysis:* You know that a distended bladder is common postpartally. You also know that pressure and trauma can reduce bladder sensitivity and tone. However, if Ms Jessup is not able to void, it may be necessary to catheterize her. You hope to avoid catheterization because of the associated risk of infection.
*Actions:* You employ nursing measures to assist Ms Jessup. You pour a measured amount of warm water slowly over her perineum while her wrist is resting in warm water. You also create a verbal picture of flowing water for her. You encourage her to use her other hand to massage her bladder.
*Analysis:* You are pleased that Ms Jessup has been able to void successfully. You decide to reassess her uterus to be certain it is now firm.
*Analysis:* The fact that Ms Jessup has been able to void two large amounts suggests that her bladder tone is adequate.
*Actions:* You tell Ms Jessup that you think she is doing well. You point out that incomplete emptying of the bladder can lead to a boggy uterus and may also contribute to the development of a bladder infection. You ask her to monitor her next two or three voidings and report to the nurse if she feels that she is not emptying her bladder fully or if she begins voiding in small amounts.

Nice job! You made accurate assessments and employed nursing actions effectively. You also treated Ms Jessup like a responsible adult by explaining the situation and involving her in assuming responsibility for her own care.

29. Inquire about her usual eating habits and provide information regarding RDA if she desires.

30. Observe how the mother interacts with others: is she animated, does she smile, does she keep eye contact, is she able to ask for what she needs, is she hesitant or reticent with you or with specific family members? Remember that many of the characteristics just listed are culturally conditioned and therefore subjective, and careful follow-up is needed.

31. (a) Episiotomy: applying cold packs, using a sitz bath, sitting on a firm surface, spraying the area with warm water after urinating. (b) Hemorrhoids: witch hazel packs, Tucks, patting when drying after urinating. (c) Afterpains: warm packs, holding pillow against abdomen, lying on her stomach, analgesics.

32. The mother wears a firm bra and avoids any stimulation to the breasts. Engorgement occurs and then will slowly dissipate. It is uncomfortable for the mother.

33. (a) Assess her steadiness, dizziness, skin temperature and characteristics, skin color, BP, and pulse. (b) Need for cleansing the vulva and perineum after voiding with a spray bottle of warm water or something similar, patting with toilet paper instead of wiping, pat from front to back to decrease incidence of UTI, any measures to increase her comfort. (c) Make sure she knows how to operate the emergency call button in the shower and stay in the room while she is in the shower. She is at the greatest risk of fainting at this time.

34. See Drug Guide: Rubella

35. Answers may include the desire for this child, her support system, methods of coping, resources, life desire, knowledge base.

36. By providing support, encouragement, and information as desired by the mother. Being a role model also is very helpful.

37. Sit down and listen to her. She is expressing feelings of sadness, frustration, and fear. Use reflective communication techniques and stay with her words. Avoid false reassurance and belittling comments. She needs to know she is being heard and understood and that these feelings are shared by many mothers.

38. Have the sibling come in for visits while in the birthing facility. Provide many opportunities for the sibling to have special attention or activities, cuddle the sibling, and introduce him/her to the new baby. Provide opportunities for caretaking and holding and introduction to the new role of big sister or brother.

39. The father or support person can be included more readily by encouraging him or her to visit whenever possible during the day or evening and to participate in infant care, encouraging him or her to come in for infant feeding, including him or her in parenting classes in the postpartal unit, being supportive of his or her efforts, providing time for any questions, including him or her in all teaching.

    These are just a few possibilities. You may have thought of others.

40. You should include information about her obstetric history, including the following: number of pregnancies, births, and abortions; significant prenatal problems and conditions; date and time of birth; medications given (anesthesia and analgesics); course of labor and birth (e.g., time of rupture of membranes, use of forceps, episiotomy, prolonged second stage); sex, Apgar score, and present condition of the infant, along with pertinent recovery room data; available support systems (in many agencies the mother's marital status has little relevance; the focus is on the support she has available to her); any existing problems or complaints (including allergies to food or drugs); method of feeding the infant; teaching needs.

    If you included most of this information, you are on the right track. If you included the physical aspects but neglected the support and teaching areas, you may find it helpful to review

material related to psychologic adjustments and teaching needs during the early postpartal period.

41. (a) High on your list of priorities in planning Carla's physical care should be rest and comfort. With an 18-hour labor, you know she has been up all night and most of the preceding day. Her third-degree extension and hemorrhoids make comfort important, and meeting this need will enable her to rest more easily.

    Because this is probably her first shower, safety is a fairly high priority, as it is with most women following birth. You should also use this time for postpartum teaching before she is discharged.

    If you listed bladder or intestinal elimination as a high priority, you may wish to review your textbook.

    It is always pertinent to assess a postpartal woman for hemorrhage, but since her fundus has remained firm, it would not be your highest priority.

    (b) You can assess Carla's attitude toward her child by unobtrusively observing her with her infant and by discussing the subject with her in an open, nonjudgmental way. Although her history suggests a possible bonding problem, it is not appropriate to jump to conclusions without further data. Frequently parents will express initial disappointment about a child's sex or behavior and then bond beautifully later.

42. Due to the incision, the mother needs careful, gentle assessment of her uterine fundus and a full surgical assessment.

43. (a) Patient-controlled analgesia is helpful for the client in that they can press the button for release of an analgesic agent as they need it for comfort. (b) The PCA pump is set to deliver a specified amount of analgesic with each push of the button.

44. See text, pp. 953–954

45. See text, pp. 954–955

46. See text, pp. 955–958

47. It is important for LaTisha to know that the test is less accurate until there is an adequate intake of breast milk or formula. Although a test will be taken before discharge, the follow-up second test is essential.

# 17 Answer Key

1. Answers include assessment, teaching, counseling.
2. Typically only one or two postpartal visits are planned, long-term follow-up is not anticipated, and the scope of the visit is focused (on postpartal needs) rather than comprehensive.
3. See text, pp. 962–963
4. Terminate the visit
5. b
6. The newborn's skull bones are soft, and permanently flattened areas may develop if the infant lies consistently in one position.
7. Answers may include the following: a side-lying position aids in drainage of mucus, decreases the risk of aspiration if the infant regurgitates, allows air to circulate around the healing umbilical cord, and is more comfortable for newly circumcised males.
8. Sponge baths are recommended until the umbilical cord has fallen off and the site has healed (about 2 weeks).
9. See text, p. 967
10. axillary
11. F
12. T
13. F
14. F
15. T
16. F
17. T
18. See text, pp. 969–970
19. Answers may include restoring her physical condition, developing competence in caring for and meeting the needs of her newborn, establishing a relationship with her new child, adapting to an altered lifestyle and family structure.
20. See text, pp. 972–973
21. 6
22. 1
23. 1
24. 1
25. 6
26. 1
27. 6
28. Answers may include failure to cuddle or soothe the infant, failure to seek eye-to-eye contact, failure to call infant by name, failure to attain adequate supplies to care for the infant, calling infant by a nickname that promotes ridicule, inadequate infant weight gain, infant dirty and poorly kept, severe diaper rash.
29. The first action would be to elicit information regarding what the mother means by "having trouble." Breastfeeding difficulties may be associated with the following: position of the baby, sore or cracked nipples, breast engorgement, and concerns regarding whether the baby is getting enough to eat. Once you have more information you can address the specific problem and provide information and support. Be sure to have community resources identified so that you will be able to assist the new family.

1. (a) Greater than 500 mL in first 24 hours after birth; uterine atony, lacerations of genital tract, retained placental fragments. (b) After first 24 hours postbirth; retained placental fragments or membranes.

2. Joan is predisposed to early postpartum hemorrhage because of overdistention of the uterus, which is present with a full-term multiple pregnancy, and because of her precipitous labor.

3. See text Figure 33–2. Answers include a slow, steady, free flow of bleeding as assessed by pad counts or weighing peri pads; boggy, soft fundus that does not stay contracted with massage and that expresses large clots; changes in vital signs that reflect possible hypovolemia.

4. The nursing diagnosis you developed, ***Potential Fluid Volume Deficit*** related to blood loss, is an important one. Joan is at risk for bleeding secondary to uterine atony. This nursing diagnosis would alert you to intervene if she demonstrates signs of early postpartal bleeding. Another possible nursing diagnosis is ***Anxiety*** related to excessive bleeding.

5. Early identification and management of uterine relaxation/atony and blood loss are high priorities. Another high priority is assisting Joan and her husband to deal with the anxiety over her bleeding.

6. a

7. Assess fundal height and firmness, administer methylergonovine maleate as ordered, have woman empty bladder frequently. If the bleeding is profuse, give oxygen by mask, give medications, and assess effectiveness. Blood loss may cause anemia, so assess for pallor and fatigue and check hematocrit. Encourage rest while facilitating maternal-infant attachment.

8. b

9. *Actions:* As you assess Carrie's episiotomy for redness, swelling, warmth, and intactness, you would also visualize and palpate her total perineal area to assess for hematoma development. *Actions:* Your nursing actions to improve comfort would include application of covered ice packs to decrease the swelling and discomfort. You may also use sitz baths to aid in fluid absorption and give analgesics as ordered and needed. You may also encourage her to void to avoid the need for catheterization. Careful observation and palpation of this site are essential so that you can assess any extension or enlargement of the hematoma. Frequent monitoring of vital signs q15min will enable you to assess any blood loss and the possible development of shock. You would also notify her physician of any increase in the size of the hematoma or changes in vital signs. Discomfort experienced by women after birth is often overlooked. By your thought processes and nursing actions, you have done much to alleviate her discomfort.

10. Two key nursing assessments that would lead you to suspect subinvolution are failure of the uterus to decrease in size at the expected rate and prolongation of lochia rubra or return of lochia rubra after the first several days of the postpartal period. Breastfeeding assists in involution, as you know, but you should not rule out the possibility of subinvolution in breastfeeding mothers if these signs exist.

11. Administer oral Methergine and antibiotics as ordered, encourage increase in fluid intake and a diet high in iron and multivitamins, do pad counts or weigh peri pads (1g = 1 mL).

12. See text, p. 988

13. d

14. c

15. a

16. See text, pp. 989–990

17. Evaluative outcome criteria would include the following: exhibits signs of wound healing, such

as decreased drainage, swelling, or redness of tissues; has a normal temperature; demonstrates increased tolerance for ambulation; understands treatment regimen, self-care, preventive measures, and implications for the care of her newborn.

Your evaluative outcome criteria may differ from these but should address some of these aspects.

18. Instruct the mother to take the entire course of prescribed antibiotics, foster rest, instruct her to avoid use of tampons or douches or having intercourse until she is told she can resume these activities, schedule a follow-up visit, encourage increased fluid intake and a diet high in protein and vitamin C.

19. Jeanne McGuire is at risk for overdistention of her bladder. Her risk factors included regional anesthesia and birth of twins (overdistention of the uterus). In addition, your physical findings that would support your response of "yes" are: the uterus is above the umbilicus and displaced to the right (by the distended bladder), and vaginal bleeding has increased because the uterus cannot contract adequately.

Initial therapy is directed toward assisting her to empty her bladder: for example, pouring warm water over the perineum; providing pain medication as needed prior to her attempt to void; and applying ice packs to the perineum immediately postpartum to minimize edema, which can interfere with voiding. If these measures don't assist Jeanne to void, then catheterization may be done.

20. Decreased bladder sensitivity resulting in an inability to empty the bladder and bladder distention, normal postpartum diuresis, and possible bladder trauma because of the birth process.

21. Answers may include the following: Administer antibiotics and antispasmodics; monitor I & O; teach prevention by encouraging client to increase fluid intake, void after intercourse, use cotton crotch underwear; and teach proper perineal hygiene.

22. Traumatized tissue: fissured or cracked nipples; overdistention: milk stasis.

23. Answers may include fever; chills; malaise; tachycardia; headache; flulike symptoms; and warm, reddened, painful areas.

24. Analgesics for discomfort, antibiotics, bed rest, increased fluid intake, supportive bra, frequent feeding of baby.

25. See text, p. 998

26. Answers may include increased amounts of clotting factors; presence of normal postpartal thrombocytosis; release of thromboplastin substances from tissues of decidual, placental, and fetal membranes; increased amounts of fibrinolysis inhibitors.

27. a

28. b

29. a

30. c

31. c

32. b

33. b

34. a

35. Instruct the woman to avoid prolonged elevation of legs in stirrups, avoid knee gatch on beds, avoid leg crossing. Encourage early ambulation, regular leg exercises after cesarean birth, walking, use of support hose, increased fluid intake.

36. Provide comfort measures, maintain heparin therapy, monitor for signs of pulmonary embolism, instruct client to avoid standing for prolonged periods and crossing legs.

37. b

38. c

39. Protamine sulfate

40. b

41. See text, pp. 1001–1004: Critical pathway, discharge planning/home care section.

42. See text, p. 1004